A SEASON OF MISTS

MYRNA BROWN

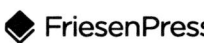 FriesenPress

Suite 300 - 990 Fort St
Victoria, BC, V8V 3K2
Canada

www.friesenpress.com

Copyright © 2016 by Myrna Brown
First Edition — 2016

All rights reserved.

No part of this publication may be reproduced in any form, or by any means, electronic or mechanical, including photocopying, recording, or any information browsing, storage, or retrieval system, without permission in writing from FriesenPress.

ISBN
978-1-4602-8744-6 (Hardcover)
978-1-4602-8745-3 (Paperback)
978-1-4602-8746-0 (eBook)

1. FAMILY & RELATIONSHIPS, DEATH, GRIEF, BEREAVEMENT

Distributed to the trade by The Ingram Book Company

For Juli —
a beautiful woman
nurse

Dedication

Denis

Myrna Brown

Acknowledgments

Michal, Denis, Bear, John, Terri, all my family and friends
who continue to encourage and support me as I write.
Those who believe love is not a myth and have
courageously set sail for its shore.
Those for whom devotion is not a duty but a privilege.
Those who achieved loving and grieve still for a dear one's presence.
Those who remember well and are propelled forward by memory and are
confident that memory will light their path and enhance their future.

Autumn, 2000
Central Coast, Oregon
Belle Haven

> She was alone and still, gazing out to sea; and when she felt his presence and the worship of his eyes her eyes turned to him in quiet sufferance of his gaze, without shame or wantonness.
>
> —*James Joyce, a Portrait of the Artist as a Young Man*

From shore to shore

The vestiges of a spider web cling to the screen on the porch where she sits, and in the dark center a dead insect blows back and forth in the light breeze like a luffing sail. The deserted web doesn't let go even in a gust. Not until spring will it let loose, and that will be under the strength of an uneasy, rain-whipping wind. For now, it lifts and floats, and she catches it in the corner of her eye, like a living thing. She's alone.

The sting of death, his presence gone, the shadow of widowhood… nothing she has read or experienced over the years resonates with her anguished response to losing Da.

Fog has settled in, and today, not even the blush of the afternoon sun diffuses the light. She doesn't know the time of day, only that it's cold and she should turn on the furnace or build a fire. It's getting past the time she might have read on the porch with a cup of tea, the time of day he might have been at his desk writing to family. As if entrapped by his death in a cold, dark cavern, she has had no escape from the all-consuming mist that whispers around her.

Her fear of her death had stirred in her a need to sacrifice, "Not to die, not to die, not to die," she nearly chanted. When Matthew was taken, she no longer crucified herself. Whatever debt was owed, she had paid. Now the altar was bloodied again without her concession, and she hid in the foggy shadows to obscure the face of God.

No act upon any altar would wake him. Possibly, he had sacrificed his integrity but not to God, not to stave off death or to guarantee life hereafter. Rather, he sought to experience the present, aspiring always to love, to be loved, to give and receive, to acquire knowledge and flood his senses with worldly pleasures. Devotion to her was one of his deepest pleasures.

They had chosen this bungalow on the beach near a small coastal town not long after they became lovers because it provided the setting for the kind of intimacy they had grown into, a way of loving that they thought was apart, something spiritual, and if not, close to it. Distinct and different from other couples, they believed their kind of loving was something significant to be celebrated in some safely remote place, like a home by the sea: like Belle Haven.

They came to love the mornings of settled-in fog, the cover of cloud, much like the late afternoon opaqueness that she is experiencing now, a metaphor to them then, surrounding and hiding them as it often did, surreally filling their senses, separating them from any other time or place. It was then the mist might begin to vanish like the spirit of a hesitant ghost.

Bright, blue days would break over the treacherous ocean, untamed and turning the waves from gray to the deepest of transparent greens, jade-like and translucent. From their glassed porch, they had often waited for the transformation from a foggy day to bright sunlight, when, like an apparition, the constant tides would reappear below them, washing into the coves, gushing foam that arced and flashed in the air. The light glanced off the breaking waves and tunneled through, defeating the mist; and the irrepressible colors, from the wet gray of the sand to the wandering, scuttling clouds in the blue sky, bore through. The dark mossy cliff they called their "half a mountain," a high, forested escarpment to the south, would be suddenly glorious like velour, a set, as if it were staged for the opening curtain.

Finally, since they married ten years before, their hideaway had become their permanent home. Every day, every hour the view toward the sea changed. They were addicted to it; it drew them. After the beauty of the Louvre in Paris, after the Rijks in Amsterdam, or the canals of Venice, the Prado in Madrid or after Gaudi's otherworld cathedral in Barcelona, their home was still a wonder to them and seemed to welcome them back: a package on the stoop; a NYT Sunday edition their friend Frank had forgotten to pick up; the red camellias rusting but hanging on; gardenias the white of snow; or the slick, orange petals of the begonias in full bloom; rosebushes that needed to be cut back.

To reestablish themselves and to make it feel like home again they performed insignificant minor tasks, like righting a crooked watercolor, or replacing a bulb. The fire was laid. The desk was opened, the pen refilled, and artifacts the cleaning people had moved were put in place. Even the seascape before them would seem to have changed, distinguished perhaps by new driftwood on the shoreline or by some tangled tree root having shifted up snug against a dune.

Da would sit on their glassed-in porch, the sea before him, succumbing to the warmth ploughing through the broken clouds. While dozing, he may have spun the whole cloth of a dream with infinite detail, some bizarre story with a hopeless beginning and tragic end. Sometimes it seemed to him as though he were a participant. In others he was a spectator, simply a witness. It was as if while he looked on, a mad genius other than himself was inside his brain, someone able to fabricate visions, grotesque or beautiful; objects he'd never seen; colors in an unnatural spectrum; texture he'd not experienced; high temperatures and low; dark and light. He may have been swept along in a strong current or held pinned down to the ground in the midst of chaos. He may have run across barren fields. He might have experienced opiate-like dreams of bliss or the angst of a lost child.

As with all who dream, only remnants of the images remained, perhaps some ribbing, useless swatches and snipped off bits of scrap to prove that such extraordinary events could have transpired in his sleeping brain. The feelings when he wakened lasted far longer than the dreams, which seemed frustratingly incoherent upon recall, bereft of their magic, significance and complicity. The little fabric left was unfit to stitch together a recounting.

Da may have tried to patch together such a dream for her before it slid quickly into oblivion, especially when he was left with the residual feelings stirred in him, that mysterious emergence of a feeling for which there is nothing to explain, unless it *be* the dream. A sad dream may have shadowed him, and to shirk it, he might have attempted to describe its pattern, wanting to be rid of the untraceable feelings it had evoked, those unsettling feelings that last far longer than the dream he couldn't divine.

Sometimes, she may have been involved in her painting, alone in her own world. His favorite, the one picture he asked her not to sell, was of the small harp-shaped cove from where it was his habit to fish. Just above it, a large flat stone extended part way over the cove, and sometimes provided him shelter in a hard rain if he moved in under it. He was inured to the drizzle and could fish long into the mornings. Suzan and Da used the same stone to stand above the cove and enjoy a high tide. The waves would tumble in and nearly reach their sandaled feet as they expanded their lungs and breathed in the salty spray, tasting it on their lips and tongue.

When he roused, not to interrupt, he might have written her snatches of his thoughts, inspired by her, his muse, he said, and sometimes his hand slid across the page covering it with endearments, or perhaps describing how he saw her chin tilt a certain way when she was assessing the effect of her last brushstroke, how she stood on one foot, holding one hand out, to lean in close to the canvas. He loved her.

The white oak interior contrasts with his mahogany desk, an antique, and the centerpiece of the sprawling room. Two matching ginger jars sit atop it, and a plant trails low between them. Behind it hangs a December, 1997 poster from an exhibit in Amsterdam at the Rijks Museum: *Langs Velden en Wegen*, chosen not just as memorabilia or for its beauty, but because one of the three riders sits on his horse exactly as Suzan's father had; the crook of his arm, the black hat he wore, so like him in his purposeful way of striding ahead, taking the lead. They framed the print rendered in tones of green and blue and gray in a wooden frame the color of antique pewter.

"I never knew your father. Am I like him?"

"Very much." She held her feelings about her father close and responded no further.

Da's self-expression in his writing was equivalent to her painting. It was his art. Lifting the lid of the great desk, pulling out the writing table, Da would settle into the chair, his ink bottle to his right and his yellow legal pad or sometimes his personal stationery, often partially filled with his highly stylized script. He wrote letters to his four children and five grandchildren, maybe a letter or a note to her as if she were absent when she was making art, as indeed she sometimes was.

Her favorite chair looked to the sea, and she might read or cross-stitch as he wrote prolifically; she let him be in another place and time. It was not necessary to them to fill a silence. They both read often, and he read several books in random fashion, leaving them about. He had favorites with notes in the margins blazing the trail his mind took.

If the temperatures were warm, they could open the windows. They might have planned their winter trip to the Spice Islands on such a day, a languid, peaceful place where the locals harvest nutmeg and braid their hair with colorful beads, someplace where the sunlight was dependable and no mist crept in overnight. They had a love-hate relationship with the Oregon coast's near-constant mantle of fog during this season, the half-hearted rains. But Belle Haven was home. The climate was unlike any other climate they had known, and sometimes the weather was a match for their more melancholic moods. They might have escaped by going west into the expanse of the Willamette Valley to find a small winery or by going south along the Rogue River for their favorite Rogue blue cheese, darkly veined and creamy. It didn't crumble on a cracker, he remarked when later they enjoyed it before the fire.

They might have walked a ways in the woods above them, delighted to see a native Oregon Silverspot alight on a meadow violet, and they might have sat on the trunk of a downed tree to watch the rare butterfly hover, powered by paper-thin wings as it fed. They might have scaled to the top of the escarpment on a trail they themselves had worn, where, looking down at Belle Haven, they might have remarked on the bald eagle's spectacular view. The eagle may have been lifted by a current they couldn't feel and vicariously they may have felt its wings expand. They would have been quiet, listening to the sound of the leaves rustling beneath their feet. They might have locked arms above the coves, the majesty of the ocean like make believe far beneath them. They might have carried the picnic basket, and the chill would have still been on the wine.

The leaves – orange, red, yellow, green in early fall – stacked like paper on each other, not yet mulched by the rain, and they would have seen their imprints and heard the leaves reshuffling as they retraced their steps. The bared deciduous trees among the young pines would have allowed the autumn sun to slip through the diverging shadows and crisply light the leafy floor of the forest.

They were drawn by their unspoken need to be within touching distance. Their companionship was not passive, not a routine they had fallen into. Rather, they lived purposefully for the other, and the days seemed lengthened for them, as they lived them to the full with awareness and gratitude. This was how their days were, whether in companionship or in solitude; they were as steadily content as humans can be for the most part, neither habitually in ecstasy or agony, but knowing the reaches of each, having experienced the wonder and fatigue of life's push and pull.

Today, the day of his death, the misty curtain won't be parted by the wind or vanquished by the warm rays of the sun. The sun won't appear like the magic that his presence was.

Left and south, the rocky crags jut out, altering the shoreline, and the Pacific seems to turn upon itself, churning with incongruent and opposing tides. When they walked the shore they were careful of these tides, not to be cut off from home. The coastline runs directly north to south except for the rocky detours it makes around the steep lava deposits, those molten, flaming rivers that stretched centuries past into the cooling water, slowing, taking shape, mounding and thinning, leaving curious coves like open shells or abandoned shelters, changing the very bed of the sea. The lava must have been a great interruption, destroying some of the habitats while introducing others, like the tide pools they stepped over, encrusted with rough, tenacious barnacles. Naturally, there were winners and losers of such catastrophic change. One species is snuffed and another conceived, surely acts of God.

She turns, and the familiar edges of the cliffs are obscured. She sees only a hint of the stand of Sitka spruce, gnarled and shaped by the salt and wind. They stand like silk-screened shadows, their trunks bent; some broken down upon themselves, no longer limber enough to sway, having lent their graceful stature to the northern winds long ago. On this day, with only a slight breeze, the stand of old-growth timber holds hazy poses like dancers on a darkened stage.

Everything she sees is gray without color, and, like gauze, the mist seems to cover a great wound. She can't see the surf surging and scrubbing clean the beach, perpetually etching wide semi-circles in the sand.

Sounding a course

A distant foghorn penetrates, low and somber, repeating. A more distant horn answers: three long monotone mournful blasts. She feels the sound in her stomach, a wounding echo, reminding her she is lost, lost without him.

But, like that ship's horn, maybe other familiar sounds will help her locate her inner self in this vastness of grief and bring her out of the fog of her thoughts. She stands and listens to the hum of the refrigerator, putting her cheek against the cool smoothness of the door. A single wind chime has freed itself, and its sound is harsh and toneless as it bats against the window.

She clicks on the furnace, turning the temperature to seventy-five. She'll not turn it down as they routinely do; she'll listen during the night for the warmed air rushing through the vents, adjusting to the night air. She'll hear the soft groaning of Belle Haven's supporting timbers. She'll cling to familiar sounds and not be lost. Ancient ships did that; they found their way in the night depending solely on the rebounding sounds echoing their location. Sound signals were the mariners' best friend during periods of low visibility and certainly of more assistance than groping along with only the information supplied by a lead line. She'll listen keenly to identify every sound. Why, why is Da gone?

Everything in her vision seems changed and unfamiliar, and yet it is all well-known after this decade here with Da. She has forgotten to water the indoor plants. The basil droops. She doesn't know Da's schedule for watering the orchids in the library. He even had the patience to wait nearly five years for an orchid to grow and bloom. How long will it be before the orchids are affected by his absence? She doesn't answer the seemingly incessant ringing phone. She feels her tremulous heart, the fear-induced increase of her pulse as she looks Da's death face on.

She tries to nap, but not in their bed. She goes into the guest room, where they'd never slept together, avoiding his smell, avoiding the library where his onyx-colored leather chair points west like an extension of the earth and sky. Sheet music stands open on the piano, a concerto not yet perfected. She wants none of the familiar to pierce through. Perhaps the cloud in her mind should be welcome as it gathers protectively to obscure her vision of him dead. She cannot rest.

She wanders about and wants nothing to do with things tied to him externally, nothing that pertains to him. There is no escape. She sees his hand in everything. She doesn't handle or cradle objects as one might expect, except for turning the ring she wrested from his hand, suddenly wanting some last token when they told her he was dead. She is oblivious to the hour and has no appetite. She feels restless.

Her strongest feeling past the pain is like swollen tissue surrounding a wound. In that most tender of places is the acknowledgment that she alone knows whom she lost. For the first time in her life, she wants to confide their history and receive affirmation and comfort from someone in her world. She is humbled by her unusual need to confide, having had him as her confidant. She feels friendless. The deep ruts on this path of roughshod grieving won't be graded smooth until she tells, until she can connect with someone who understands. She must not be alone. She is a danger to herself. Her respirations are irregular and her sighs are weighted with sorrow, though she has not cried tears.

She sits again, feeling with her fingers the coarse texture of the woven fabric of her chair. She rubs the smooth gold of the ring against the cloth already worn by use. The diamonds catch on the threads and aren't brilliant as they turn. Given light, the near-perfect stones gleam authentically, but the light is insufficient, and there's little reflection of their splendor.

Otherwise, she is still, and the day will continue to pass, dull and dark. It begins to drizzle, and minuscule drops collect on the skylights, brimming and trembling as they converge and trail like tears. She leans her head back to watch them quiver and combine into a ragged trickle, and she sees how rivers are made, how nature rules.

A SEASON OF MISTS

But whom can she tell? Certainly, not his children who were prone to call up memories of Cora, their deceased, adored mother, when they visited, who never knew Da had loved Suze during their childhood, through their teens, through college, into the years they began their families. To them, he was their devoted father, not an unfaithful husband.

Neither Da's children nor Suzan know of Cora's role in the resistance movement during WWII in the Netherlands. Nor did they know that Cora had literally saved Da's life after the 1940 invasion, feeding and hiding him at her own peril.

Fear and shame, a potent swill, a drink from hell. Had she known the full scope of the truth, had she seen inside the fossil, Suzan would have quit Da. Such was her nature. Respect for Cora would have demanded it, and the guilt would have overwhelmed her. As it is, she feels still the twinges of guilt for loving Da over the years he was married to Cora. Cora's death changed everything for them. Because Suzan anticipates his children coming to Belle Haven, the shame has come to the fore. Da's and her past is something to be hidden, not told. Afraid for her future, she is unable to console herself.

To Suzan, his children seemed to be a unit unto themselves even clannish when they came to Belle Haven, as they sat around an evening fire in the great room, confidants to each other. She felt detached, even from Da, as they laughed and talked among themselves. Although they appeared to care about Suzan, she knew she would never be considered his real wife; she was certainly no stand-in for their mother. She was not their flesh and blood.

His children should never know how the past had mapped Da and Suzan's future. She believes the truth would tear the thin, fragile fabric of any family, even of the most cohesive cloth. For that matter, unadulterated facts can coarsely strip a family apart for all time. His children knowing of their past would shear any attachment she had to his family's world. Because they are part of Da, she wants them in her life. Maybe his death will open their hearts to her. Belle Haven's doors are wide open to them but her trove of memories remains private to her.

Although she's unsure of her place in their minds, she also wants his children to have a legacy of trust, and wants them always to have entry to her heart and Belle Haven with its large windows looking out, the view instilling perspective and wisdom by its pure vastness.

During vacations here, on a clear night, one of the grandchildren had almost always darkened the room and pointed to the stars through the skylights.

"Grandpa, which is that one?" Daan, his namesake, might say.

"Well, Venus and Jupiter, for starters…"

"Grandpa, do you have a telescope?" Dusty had asked on one occasion. How glad Da was to answer their questions. They had gathered jackets to go outdoors into total darkness to identify the brightest stars, wondering about galaxies and constellations, the inexplicability of infinity. He taught them to reverence those moments, and to acknowledge whose hand had thrust the planets into self-spinning, expanding universes.

Someone should know

Daan's working, traveling days for the World Bank were over, having managed agricultural projects in over sixty countries, having been witness to the hungry, the wounded and the defeated spirits of the survivors of the civil wars that seemed to abound. In many of the poorest countries, fields lay fallow, which planted could bring prosperity and equality. Often there were more soldiers with guns than croppers with their hoes and seedlings. Often it was up to the women and girls to ensure a harvest.

Someone should know how well she knew his proud heart, how he would have travelled more to make the world a better place. He loved her, and their love sheltered them from these realities as, perhaps, love is meant to do. Still, he carried a burden of not leaving a less brutal world. "No one should have to go hungry in our day and time," he'd said when he spoke of the plight of the hungry. "It's a matter of distribution." And, of course, they invested in charities whose science was solid and that he had researched carefully.

After their marriage in 1990, they travelled for pleasure, always in first class. But he anchored here at Belle Haven with her like someone who had been alone and out to sea but was now returned and unready to face those hazards again.

Only she had known the depth of his sense of being alone when he was away and without her. Long ago before they married, he called her his faraway dream girl. Someone should know of their long journey, the sacred, precious path they took, perhaps profane to others had their intimacy been exposed. There seems to be no one.

She knows not to expect him through the garage door, but she does… or just out of the shower, wet and refreshed, rubbing his morning beard against her face. He lathered in a small ivory bowl he had picked up in China, and it is slightly stained where he rubbed his sable brush, leaving faint, brownish circles. Tomorrow, she will see that the ivory handle of the soapy brush still rests against the dish as he left it. On most occasions, he shaved twice, and she came to expect the freshness of his face in her neck when they cooked in the evening.

He sometimes grinned through his soaped upper lip, his eyes larger, twinkling, as if he had pulled a trick on her. He shaved with relish and enjoyment. He loved mornings, and now for her, it is becoming night, and she mustn't allow the shape of him to float even murkily through the fog of her mind. She must close her eyes, let the vagueness replace the vivid and let the darkness close in. Further out, in the open sea the foghorn repeats. She listens and closes her eyes. She fastens her feelings to the ticking clock, willing her heart to slow, breathing consciously.

The sun dissolves into the lavender stretch of the horizon, still filtering through the tinted cloth of diminishing dusk, like a seamless, crumpled robe of mauve velvet. She doesn't really prepare for bed. She'll just lie down as she is. Already, she knows she won't stay past dawn. She may as well not change into a gown. She'll not wash her face. She'll rise only to sit, but not near his chair, not with any earthly reminder of him. The phone rings again, demanding something of her she can't give.

He's stubbornly alive in her mind, and she must reconcile herself to his having left her. But, her imagination smells him, like fresh lumber, like cedar newly split, like a walk in the woods. Just as near is the memory of the wet coldness of his body as she tried to turn him in the surf. Her thoughts waver between Da being dead and Da so brilliantly alive. She must begin to substitute the memory of the living image with the memory of the collapsed figure in the cove in order to really know he is gone. But she has no control. How can he be gone?

He didn't need her care. He was strong and fit at the age of seventy-five, but he let her rub the lotion into his back, put the drops in his eyes. She loved pleasuring him. And, she did it well. His smile made his eyes transparent, like waves on the cusp of breaking. Do eyes light up? They seemed to when she turned toward him on their long walks. They seemed to when they swirled their wine and held up their glasses to see the rivulets on the glass, the "legs" of a good wine. Like sipping away at time itself, not to let it pass too quickly, they drank with appreciation and grace, judiciously selecting moments to savor a favored Pinot Noir or on occasion a Kir Royale.

Neither was good at saying goodbyes. God knows they had done it often enough. Nor did he do it well this time. He just went. She was watching him fish; he was reeling in his line, and the tide had begun filling the cove behind him. She knew he would soon be forced out, and that he would start up the path. She started coffee. Carefully, she had measured half decaffeinated and scooped the other half from a dark Kenyan roast they had found at Peets in San Francisco. Going back to the window, she saw him turn to step over the flank of the rocky formation in the small cove. He collapsed, face down. Though she didn't know, his heart had failed him. She expected him to get up and collect his fishing gear, but he didn't. He lay there, and the incoming waves washed over him, lifting and moving his body like flotsam. To retrieve him, she called for help and stumbled toward him before the tide could tug him under and away.

They were lovers, and only ten of the thirty years since their acquaintance were left to them, though they would have claimed them all were it not for those they loved in other ways, ways that matter throughout one's lifetime. But then Cora died, and it was with that heartache their chance to marry had come about.

He was flawed, she knew, to have betrayed Cora. She must have been a strong person coping with four children during his many absences. Even after having these years with him at Belle Haven, Suzan sees Cora's picture with their family in the library, and envies the years they had together as one family. She envies their wholeness. He has no other reminder of Cora's that she knows of. Still, she wants what Cora had and she did not. Her divorce from David, with all the release it brought, left a residue of loss and remorse, a forfeiture of hope for the idealized family so much a part of America's culture. She had simply chosen from the wrong bolt of cloth. The fabric had torn and couldn't be mended.

His children didn't answer the descriptive, elaborate letters he wrote. Instead, they called, and it was like a ritual they created among themselves. A letter returned by a call. A letter... a call. They checked in, even as they themselves fell into the pitfalls of middle-age, with all the turns and detours, the complex decisions and events of an average life.

Their education and strength of character buoyed them. For the most part, they loved life; they caught the waves, so to speak. The phone would be handed over to a grandchild, and they would talk of ballet lessons, basketball, football or even the European soccer teams. To Paul, his oldest son and Phillip, his youngest, he might have talked of a successful mission to East Africa, of President Clinton's debacle, of the abrupt halt of the Gulf War, or apartheid and Nelson Mandela's sacrifice. He wept when Rabin was assassinated. He and his children communicated, and they were family to each other.

Daan and Suzan thought that as a couple they were exceptional, and perhaps they were, giving themselves permission as they did to maintain and nurture their love. At some point, rather than continue to agonize about whether or not to just continue to correspond or afford themselves an affair, they opted to meet as often as possible, mostly in a place reminiscent of no place else: along the Pacific's gray shores, here at Belle Haven, a modern bungalow that he leased year-round and kept open. They could leave things, and they did: a variety of jackets, scarves, old sandy shoes, a few bottles of wine, love notes, fishing poles. She left what paintings she completed, and those she didn't, almost like testimony to their having secretly coupled here.

She had set up an art studio, and it stayed ready for her. Canvases, some empty, some complete, some only sketched in, were stacked against the walls. There was the coincidence of colors, the predominance of blues and greens, and a stark, near-titanium white to represent the ocean's spray. There were rusty-grays, umber (like pine straw), the vermillion reds and the blended purples of a sunset as it deepened its reflection on the sea. There was a dropcloth that hung over an easel, splotchy against the gray canvas with the colors of a palette, a work of art in and of itself. Sometimes the palette resembled the flannel-graphs of her years in Sunday school depicting Jesus and his disciples beside the Sea of Galilee. Somehow back then there were no primary colors. They were muted and blended.

Before they married, when they came, most often the heavy, drifting mist would be dispelled, but, oh, sometimes so late in the day. They would be called out into the changing day. They would be tempted by the breaking sky. They might have romped and played, and shouted, "I love you" over the ever present rush of the sea.

Here at Belle Haven, she had mourned for her son Matthew, wrestled with the angel of death and slept with her head on that proverbial rock, affected for life from her encounter. No ladder to heaven appeared. Her exhaustion from the sheer work of grieving had left her more consciously mortal, and for a time her spirit lay crumpled to what seemed to be the cold ground of his grave. She could only depend on the memory of her muscles to live out a day. Da's comfort was not enough. She lay in a ball then, as she will again now, sustaining the blows of her losses, the necessary losses for which one can't prepare. At the time of Matt's death, when she was determined to move forward, she thought too little of how Ellie, her daughter, must have felt. Instead, Suzan modeled stoicism and returned to work soon after, robot-like in her movements. *Ellie is apart but strong,* she thought.

During the years Da and Suze waited and could only be together when secreted away, they reconciled themselves to living double lives. Even so, here, they could walk in the village, look in the shops on Main Street or dine at Ernie's for cheeseburgers that their diets forbade. Arthur, the grocer, ordered them truffles from season to season and the jam they liked. He also delivered when she called in ahead, tucking things away for them before their arrival. He always selected from the best vegetables and fruits. He chilled the champagne.

At Belle Haven, all the rules went away, and they exposed themselves to the strong, unpredictable weather of passion. They were not vague in any way toward the other. In clear light, they held the hope, the hope for the gift of time. She forgave his infidelity and was complicit in their escapes together, because he meant the world to her, and she believed no other could do. She had given him entry into nearly all the places of her being.

Now, after a short decade together at Belle Haven, their time is up. One of his often-read books, Bertrand Russell's essays it looks to be, is spread open and lies face down. His habit of leaving them that way weakened the bindings. She gave him bookmarks picked up from various museum shops, but he consistently broke the backs, and would leave them, several at a time, as if he didn't want to put them away, as if he hadn't quite satisfied his curiosity. She was always careful not to lose his place when she closed them.

His books were treasures, each placed in alphabetical order according to fiction or non-fiction, gardening or geography. The greater section was historical fiction. But, he could find a Baudelaire poem and often did to please her, even though he seemed quite able to recite it out of the blue in his Dutch-accented French. He quoted Kahlil Gibran; those complicated counselling phrases that bore into her. She envied his intellect and forgave his sins. He said things she had no context for, maybe about some character Shakespeare had concocted and assigned a soliloquy. If she questioned, he pulled a volume from *The Riverside Shakespeare*. At times she was impatient and wished he wouldn't give the full explanation.

He sometimes wrote to her, even though they were together, and she would find the letters near her pillow at bedtime. She read them alone, always the next morning while he made coffee. She answered them by buttering his toast and buttoning his raincoat. She unsnarled his fishing lines. She was tender toward him. She also memorized poetic portions of his notes and repeated them back to him when they made love or when they were tenderly holding the other, or surely while walking the shoreline shoulder to shoulder. She painted with the shadow of his presence.

After their marriage, touching had become very important to them, an awakened craving they indulged. They woke in the night to reach again for the other and returned to entwining themselves: she to his back or he to hers. He hadn't known he needed or wanted the constancy of this less passionate intimacy, but was very often the one to pull her toward him. As it pleased them, they sometimes allowed their shared attraction, like a strong current to carry them to another place.

After Cora died, after he grieved, and after he eventually came back to her, they purchased the bungalow. Da managed the details; it was simpler that way.

Their losses humbled them, and they revered life. They loved each other openly and proudly. Suzan's eyes were livelier, and her ideas were more spontaneous. She picked up her paints, changing her palette and painting large. Ellie finished her masters in finance and they forged a bond forgiving of their differences, out of the fire but not yet shaped.

Engulfed

Belle Haven perches on a windswept bluff, alone, over an expansive rocky cove, with smaller coves, nearly cave-like and almost enclosed. The oddly constructed house points as if it has a prow toward the sea, and overlooks those sea-carved coves. The house is rather unsheltered looking, precarious seeming, projecting as it does over the rocks, nearly shadowing the shoreline.

The weathered cedar shakes have gone gray over time, but it is a strong house, like them, and has sustained many storms. The rooms are grand and open, and the skylights refract slanting strips of light, laying stripes on the nearly nude floors and neutral furnishings. At this moment, there are no shafts of sunshine. Momentarily she feels as if the whole of it, her with it, has washed out to sea. But, bolted down with pilings thirty feet deep, she knows it will not release itself from its impenetrable rock foundation, and she huddles there as if it can protect her from the violent shock of his death. She pulls the down pillow into a ball against her breasts, attempting to soothe herself.

During those years apart, they corresponded, met together, and said awful goodbyes as if it were the end of the world, as if they would be forever lost to each other. But later, after a halting beginning at being lovers, before they married, Belle Haven held them like a steadying hand, offering them another life, even the comfort of a village. They became somewhat indifferent to the outside world, and neither was as tortured by witnessing its random horrific suffering.

They had supposed he would go first, but they couldn't bring themselves to plan for the event. The subject wasn't talked of. At fifty-five, she had thought about, but never mentioned, the near-certainty of this time when she would lose him. They knew time was a gift, and they hadn't squandered it, even though they had no warning Da would go so soon. He had done well on the treadmill when last he saw his cardiologist. He had been given the "all clear" to exert himself.

Their beach walks were lengthy and extended around the great igneous rock slides of the Paleocene Age, and they had to step over the protruding traces of black lava in the sand. But now, he has died mid-stride. He had always measured his long strides for her to keep up until now. He has "gone ahead", as people often say, as if there is someplace to go. She wants to follow him. Why is she still here? She can almost see the imprint of his steps in the sand leading out to sea. He didn't mean to die, but she blames him from some inner place.

Tomorrow she will prepare the guest room for Ellie, but tonight she sleeps there, fitfully, alien to her surroundings, shifting to squeeze the down comforter against her whole body as if he were there. She sleeps in her clothes. She listens for the furnace to click on. She strains to hear the ticking of the old clock on the mantel in the next room. How can she bear this loss?

Unlike Da's own more graceful death, Cora's was a strenuous, ugly death, extended by all sorts of prescriptions and hopeful treatments. Da hadn't wished for Cora's death, not until the end time, when she pleaded with her eyes to be relieved of having to live it out. At that moment, he sat by her, in the company of his sons and daughters and the children, one who was too young to understand her preoccupied, subdued parents. But, they, too, stood around the room as they anticipated the death of their grandmother, and they silently cried in the company of their grandfather and their parents when they heard her last rattling breath, a deep and final sigh. Quietly, they were family to each other. Her children let go her mottling hands, placing them on her chest, leaving her side to comfort him, who was the more distraught because of his guilt.

He wept and was held by his children and their children. They held each other, and it was a kind of holding that only transpires when family members believe in each other and love deeply, when the fabric holds and no wrongdoing or betrayals have ravaged the whole. It was then he drew a punishing curtain of solitude around himself that he didn't draw open, not to them and not to Suzan, for several months. She doesn't know if he wrote a journal during that period. That span of time is lost to her. She can only know her own pain of separation and guilt. She bore the guilt with him. So much did they want each other.

A SEASON OF MISTS

The memorial service was punctuated with references to their strong family, to Cora as mother and grandmother. She was their rock, they said, nowhere more respected than in her own home. The personal tributes from the children were celebratory and long. Even her split pea soup was mentioned. She had few close friends. But for his colleagues, the small chapel in the funeral home was not nearly filled.

Because he loved Suzan and craved to be with her, Da blamed himself for Cora's death, as if by hoping for time with Suzan he had caused it. For those months, he grieved alone, unable to absolve himself, castigating himself day after day. He had wanted Suzan, his Suze, beyond measure, and regrettably, he saw himself, arrogantly, profanely godlike, causing Cora's demise at sixty-six.

He wouldn't spare himself the guilt-laden grief, and when it engulfed him without reprieve, and he was caught unawares, he sought solitude. Even these years later he had succumbed to the kind of isolation that comes of being unforgiving of one's own self, as did she. Given their life experiences, intermissions of their connectedness were unavoidable, and they prized their intimacy more acutely than they might have otherwise.

Although they were alike in that way, the gaps in their fellowship were short. They were coupled but separate, as the Prophet Gibran had recommended:

> Let there be spaces in your togetherness, and let the winds of the heavens dance between you. Love one another but make not a bond of love: Let it rather be a moving sea between the shores of your souls. Fill each other's cup but drink not from one cup. Give one another of your bread but eat not from the same loaf. Sing and dance together and be joyous, but let each one of you be alone, Even as the strings of a lute are alone though they quiver with the same music. Give your hearts, but not into each other's keeping. For only the hand of Life can contain your hearts. And stand together, yet not too near together: For the pillars of the temple stand apart, and the oak tree and the cypress grow not in each other's shadow.

For a time, when he returned to her after Cora's death, he was impotent. She thought of it as a carryover from those months that led up to and after Cora's death. The moment would come in their lovemaking – he would go slack in her hand, and cry out, "No, no." She had encouraged him to please her as he always had, bringing her to orgasm. His silent frustration disallowed her speaking of it. Sometimes his sleep was fitful and she couldn't hold him as she wished. The yearning to hold him never went away. It was an eternal flame that fed off her soul.

They went to Paris to a tiny, old-fashioned apartment, chosen for its location, let to them by a shriveled old woman, thin with silvery folds of wrinkled skin under her chin and around her neck. She was bent at the waist, her shoulders stooped, no taller than a ten-year-old. Her face seemed to hold the permanently wrinkled imprint of the resolute, those whom one sees as having become resigned to their station in life, whatever suffering it delivers. Her slim hands had tracks of deep purple, bulging veins and were pocked with red splotches owing to the fragile capillaries of the old. The thin skin of her hands shone like sheer wax paper as she pulled the door open to the small elevator.

It was evening when they arrived. They could smell that someone in another flat was cooking; it was a welcoming smell, like beef bourguignon. Later they found a small enamel pot in the oven and enjoyed it with the crusty bread they tore apart with their hands.

The old woman had also left a bottle of Veuve Cliquot champagne sitting on the small round table. The duvet was already turned down. They cranked open the window, and as they leaned out toward the red, green and blue tower twinkling in the December night, Suze turned, receiving his kiss, then receiving him. He had returned to her. Like Botticelli's Venus, being born surrounded by angels, coming out from her shell; likewise he came out of his self-imposed shell, and their fantasies took them into new, transcending realms. They heard the old woman's chair scrape across the floor above, perhaps from table to desk.

The old woman was not hard of hearing, and she winked at them and fussed about when she brought the coffee and croissants in the morning. One could hear the dishes rattle as she cautiously placed the tray with shaking hands. On the tray was the smallest of red roses. A petal fell and cupped. Later that day, they muffled their sounds but were just as successful.

Riptides

Ellie, Suzan's only daughter, arrives from San Francisco at Belle Haven in early afternoon. Ellie doesn't love many, but she loved Da. She has come both to mourn and to comfort. She doesn't know her mother's long history with him, but she and Da had come easily together after he and Suzan married.

She is looking in the refrigerator when she says, "Mom, let's go to Ernie's for dinner. Let's get out a bit. I want to talk – about how you're doing and what you want to do now that Da is gone – just talk."

Suzan looks at her tall daughter, thirty-one, a bank executive, who dresses smartly and outdoes her peers in nearly every way. She has her father's stature. She drove herself at university to get the highest grades, rarely dating, staying single and childless. She has no love life, as far as Suzan knows. In this moment, Suzan sees the little girl she had been, and momentarily it is as if Ellie's silent tears are for a broken toy or last year's rusty skates instead of another death. She's beginning to see this tall brunette as a woman, as an equal in their womanhood. Neither she nor Ellie can acknowledge or abide the largeness of Da's absence. The fact of his death fills the room.

"Cereal is all I want this evening,"

"There's no milk, Mom."

In times past, Ellie has vacationed in late summer when one could hope for a stronger sun to outdo the dense fog by mid-morning. Da and Ellie had often huddled together over the daily crossword puzzle, dallying the mornings away with their coffee. He was not paternal. They seemed to share in an easy fashion the topics that came up.

Contemplative but charismatic, they were alike in Suzan's mind. Seeing them together, loving the two of them was nearly painful. She remembers he had roughed Ellie's hair after losing to her at Scrabble.

In the past, Ellie had biked in the mornings, her lean, strong shoulders bent over the handlebars, gliding down the curves of the driveway, cycling more deeply into the fog overlaying the village. Flushed and sweaty, she might have brought back something from Rosie's, the village bakery – a Danish, a Bear's Claw – but for Da, always the cream filled profiterole. Sometimes she held a fistful of beach daisies.

But it is fall, and the sun hides. Da is gone. Hoping for a bright day might be like an unbeliever hoping to be swept away in the Rapture, or the Second Coming. The Oregon coast is like that, undiscovered by most, unless sunshine is predicted. Then people of all sort parade to the beach, disturbing the dunes, not understanding the nature of their environment, not grasping the overwhelming beauty of the overcast beaches, naked of tourists, when the paths among the dunes are as unknowable as Venice. With or without witnesses, the surf pounds; the winds rake; steady driving rains pelt; and random high tides change and rearrange the dunes like a determined deity on the sixth day.

Ellie goes to the store, and when the door closes, Suzan is caught unexpectedly in a storm of grief. She no longer has the retreat of the guest bedroom. She can't bear to go to her own room. She goes instead to the glassed porch and sits, her head buried in her hands, her first blinding tears since she hadn't saved him coming suddenly in a torrent, like rage. She wails with no one to hear, sucked under by the initial, billowing wave of grief.

Finally, still groaning, she calms and opens the door to their bedroom for the first time since he went. It is there, undisturbed, readied for them, his scents released and taunting her, she splays across the bed. She wraps her face with her arms; she curls to her side; she sweeps her hands through her hair. In her anger, she feels no urge to pray; she isn't seeking grace for the hour, neither pity for her pain. She is swept under

Suzan buried her son, Matthew, in 1985. It was such a senseless death, the impaired driver crossing the line, colliding with Matt at nineteen, leaving blood, grief, brokenness and conflict. Now, she cries again for him, and the vision of his nineteen-year-old broken body looms in her face. Her losses parade before her: her mother, father, aunt, brother.

She cries for her aborted child, Da's child, of whom no one knows. At thirty-eight, after she and Da began seeing each other more often; it hadn't occurred to her that she might become pregnant. David, her first husband, had had a vasectomy, and for many years they hadn't paid any attention to her monthly cycle, which had become irregular anyway. She had assumed Da had also had the procedure and was unable to make her pregnant. In those waning years of her own fertility she forgot entirely that she might be at risk.

The shock. It was September, 1982. Ellie, at thirteen, was on the cusp of navigating through her teens. She needed her mother to be strong and emotionally healthy. She herself had many emotions to resolve. Matt had his permit and was learning to drive. Life was changing for each of them. A child would have pummeled them into a financial crisis.

Suzan had gone to a drugstore outside her neighborhood to purchase the test. She had leaned against the wall of her bathroom, hands over her eyes, saying, "Oh, God, *no!*"

Her hands had shaken when she punched in the number to call Dr. Sipes, the gynecologist who had delivered Matthew, asking for the earliest possible appointment. The receptionist could only give her an appointment a week away. Suzan had told her, "It's an emergency. I'm pregnant. I need something sooner."

There was no earlier time available, and she lived for a week with the awareness she couldn't preserve or provide for his child.

On the cold table in the chilly room, her legs in the metal stirrups, Dr. Sipes, thinking she was still married to David, had chided her, saying, "You should be spanked." He listened and palpated, measured her stomach and slid open her vagina with a stainless steel device.

"Everything looks good. If the nausea doesn't subside, call me and we'll try some medication. Drink a lot of fluids. In the meantime, use Mylanta for the acid reflux. Dry soda crackers before you get out of bed might help. We'll do amniocentesis down the road a little."

"Dr. Sipes," she had said, "I don't want this baby. I'm single now."

She had begun to shake with cold, and the nurse had put on an extra loosely knit blanket. Her angled, blue-paper covered feet protruded and seemed colder by comparison. She slipped both hands over her stomach, wanting to warm them; she also wanted to hold her fertilized womb. How could she let go of what was there, something living, something of Da implanted and conjoined in her womb?

Dr. Sipes had stood back, his large meaty hands on his padded hips. His face, nearly always cheerful, was grave. He unbuttoned the coat over his stomach and put a hand on his hip. The years had gone by, and his belt hung below his belly.

"Meet me in my office," he said.

Suzan retched yellow bile from the depth of her stomach into a kidney shaped, stainless-steel container. Not waiting until she finished, he stepped out, closing the door.

The nurse had removed the stirrups and was helping Ellie up, when she said, "He doesn't believe in doing abortions."

Her heart sinking, she had gone to sit in his office. She remembers the books on his shelves were in disorder, and various examination sheets and letters lay about. He had pushed some materials about a Planned Parenthood clinic in San Jose toward her.

Hunching over, still chilled, she had asked, "Isn't there someone local here in Santa Cruz?"

"None that I would recommend," he had said gruffly.

Her heart was torn. She had never felt so alone. She would never tell Da. There was no one. This was to become her lifelong secret. How tired she was of secrets.

The most humiliating part had to be that when she went to make arrangements she was counselled by women younger than she who were adamant that she should keep the baby. At least give her or him up for adoption, they said. They showed her pictures of tiny fingers and toes. Later, she listened to the detectable, intent little heart as the nurse performed the sonogram. The clearly audible 'swish swish' made her own heart stop. After she made the appointment for the abortion procedure and was leaving, the same group outside called out, "Don't you know you're killing a person? It's a sin against God."

Death will mock you, if you let it, showing you visions of an inevitable future when all is lost. It will hold up a record of your misdeeds. It will lure you into its shadow and feed you hard facts and bits of reality. It will make appealing the gall in its glass. Drawn and quartered, you'll lie ever so still, no longer able to feel the pain of remorse or the joy of gladness. Someday, your grave will go untended.

Suzan became suicidal before the abortion. She wanted to die along with the child she was aborting. She could easily crash the little sports car on one of the long swerving curves over the Santa Cruz Mountains. It happened all the time, someone running into the center guardrail. A barrier had been erected just so there would be no gruesome head-on collisions like in times past.

She could swim too far into Monterey Bay and let the currents sweep her under, beyond where the young lifeguards could see. There were always riptides. It had to be an accident. She wanted her shame to go with her to her grave.

But on the scheduled day of the abortion she drove herself safely to the clinic in San Jose. She walked through a group mingling in the parking lot, their signs swaying, shouting scriptures, obsessed by their cause. She walked through a corridor of hard core pro-lifers lining the sidewalk to the double door entry.

Because of the sedation she would receive, she had been instructed to bring someone to drive her home, but she had determined to do it alone. No one cleared her way, and those around her spoke in a near snarl directly in her face. Someone stood in front of her blocking the handle. She pushed the sign for those handicapped, and the obnoxious chap was taken off guard.

Sleepy, and sedated, she felt the suction, the sudden wrenching as the fetus was aspirated. She hardly bled. The immediate embryonic pain in her spirit couldn't be suctioned away. The bleeding of her soul would never stop. Maybe she could touch the hem of His garment and be healed. There was that hope or was it all a myth?

She would have been able to leave, but her blood pressure was abnormally low. The intravenous fluids were increased. They waited. By then the nurses had asked about the person who had accompanied her. Suzan turned away from the harsh lights and faced the green wall, rearranging the skimpy cotton gown. They pulled her curtain.

Knowing she was alone, they would not release her even when her blood pressure stabilized and became somewhat normal. It was late evening. There was a shift change, a long lapse and much discussion about her status.

An older more persuasive nurse, rather squat, with gray permed hair, not wearing the teddy-bear printed smock, thank goodness, very sure of herself, swiped the curtain open. "Shall we call a taxi?"

Because there was no one else, Suzan called Dr. Evans and his wife, the people in the home above her apartment from whom she rented, knowing as a physician, he would keep her confidence.

They consented to drive over the hill from Santa Cruz to San Jose, not asking any questions. They had prepared a place in the back seat of their Lincoln with a pillow and blanket. How kind they were. She gave way to the momentum of the long curves and dozed, the blanket pulled to her chin. They led her to her bed. Cathy made tea. The room was half lit from the garden lights, welcoming. Bill took her blood pressure and listened to her heart. He asked about the bleeding. For several days, she hid from the world. Their kindness had saved her. Her children coddled her. Matt and a friend retrieved the car. He made his favorite macaroni and cheese. Ellie bought frozen yogurt. Suzan hid her tears.

No one will ever know of Da's baby. She had chosen names: Jessica or Joshua. Which one had she killed? It would be her private, untreated pain. Secrets and sins are woven into the cloth of every human story, and she is no different.

Now, in the present, while Ellie is gone to the store, Suzan remembers how she craved to die rather than face the elective grief of giving up a child. This present grief of losing Da is guiltless and of a different nature, but she is enticed by death all the same, to be out of this world, to have a final release. At least Da hadn't been seduced by death. He had no thoughts like she is having now; he was not enticed to leave of his own volition. She forbids her death wish, but the dank, earthy cavern is dark, and she finds no way out.

An image of a fearfully turbulent ocean sweeps into her mind. She feels pulled under by a second undulating strong current that won't loosen her. Before she can ideate how she might take her own life, the riptide releases her, and she realizes that it is Ellie who should be told that she, Suzan, during the time she was single, a divorcee, bereft of her only son, her parents both gone, has been loved by Da all along.

She sits up. She feels strengthened knowing she will tell Ellie that she and Da had been lovers long before they married. Ellie is a woman now who can bear truths. Da had been Suzan's tether to this earth during those years when teens, growing into adulthood heartlessly leave you, when loneliness smolders like a dampened fire. Ellie is back now, emotionally with her as an adult, physically here at Belle Haven for her. It's Ellie she should tell.

This, the highest tide of grief, will subside intermittently and flush the beaches of her soul leaving the temporary patterns only nature conjures. She must avoid thinking or wishing for her own demise and steel herself against following Da. She needs the comfort that Ellie is offering. Will she be alienated or received?

Mooring

When the garage opens, Suzan startles with a lurch of hope. It's Da coming in. Ellie, loaded down with bags, sees her mother's disappointed face, flushed and swollen, but makes no comment. She carries in a hefty order: ground beef, kidney beans, cilantro, avocados, jalapeños, tortilla chips, bags of groceries. She's also found a new rosemary plant. She brings basil in a packet and tiny tomatoes and small balls of submerged mozzarella, new potatoes that need to be scrubbed.

Arthur caters to those who have vacation homes in the vicinity, and his produce is fresh and beautifully displayed. He had recognized Ellie and asked about Suzan while Ellie chose among the fruit. "She's just really in shock," Ellie had answered.

As she thanked him for loading the trunk of the hatchback rental, he had patted the car, bending, saying, "We're all in shock. Me, I feel I lost a good friend, a mighty fine man. You tell Suzan our thoughts are with her, with you both. I can deliver some groceries if you need. I expect people will be coming in. Just give me a call when you need something. I'm always here."

Da had called him "circus friendly", but Ellie saw a tear in his eye.

Now, she remembers and says, "Arthur sends his condolences, Mom."

Ellie returns to the car and carries in more bags, beginning to place the produce into the lowest drawer of the fridge. Intently, no longer immobilized, as if her tears had restored her, Suzan empties the tall, brown bags onto the pale granite. Obviously, Ellie has planned for several large meals. Suzan folds the bags and presses each one flat, opens the door to the pantry and squeezes them in between the others. The slightly soft avocados go onto the granite windowsill. Functioning, she arranges the fruit in a bowl, laying the bananas on top of the red Delicious apples.

"I bought fresh halibut. How would that be with some rosemary-garlic new potatoes for this evening?" She looks up from her crouched position in front of the refrigerator.

"Whatever you plan, Ellie…"

Ellie stands, the fridge door open behind her. They must talk at some point about their loss, about what her mother will do. She feels alone in her responsibility to console or give any kind of guidance. She misses who Matt might have been as an adult, an older and perhaps wiser brother. Will her mother stay alone here in Belle Haven? How best to comfort her, when she, too, is feeling the magnitude of their loss?

"Mom, is there anything I can…?

Rather than answer Ellie's unfinished question, Suzan leaves the kitchen to stand before the great windows of the sun porch, her back to Ellie; she shakes her head no. She feels as if she has collapsed on the shore. Yet another wave rolls over her.

She doesn't know where to begin. Her arms are wrapped around herself, and she rocks from back to front. She rubs her colorless lips together, sucking them in. They have begun to chap. By tomorrow, they will swell, and she'll apply an ointment. Her tongue, once attracted, plays unconsciously with the tiny, raw cracks, and her lips will remain chapped and sore for more than a week. As she gazes out, righting herself, she believes she may be a step closer to releasing some of the truth to Ellie.

Late evening as they prepare for bed, Ellie puts on a blue, plaid, flannel shirt, worn at the cuffs, the collar nearly threadbare. "You need a robe. I'll get you one. Hold on…"

Suzan returns to Ellie's room with a long gown and matching robe. Pale saffron, she runs her hand down its silk, satin-like front, smoothing it, handing it to Ellie on the hanger. "Mom, this is too good. You know what a rough sleeper I am."

Ellie slips just the robe over her flannel shirt. The effect is ridiculous, and Suzan laughs. Suddenly they are laughing and crying at once. They hold each other, and Suzan's tears come freely and warmly now, spreading into a circle on the shoulder of the robe that Ellie wears. Suzan's sobs are without the anger, without the keening. She takes comfort in Ellie's presence.

"Oh, Ellie, it's so good you're here. Thank you for coming."

"Mom, I wouldn't be anywhere else." Ellie turns away from their embrace, blows out a deep breath and both fists go to her eyes.

Suzan reaches to comfort her daughter out of habit, drawing Ellie's arms down away from her eyes. "Cry, Ellie. It's no good to hold back."

Suzan dresses for sleep in a slim fitting black silk, a gift from Da many years before. It is her first night back in their bedroom, her first night there without Da to slide his hand down the back of her gown. "Rubenesque," he described her. He liked the curve of her back. He loved softness and texture.

Alongside his inhaler, a book, *The Thorn Birds,* lies face down on his bedside table. She marks the place and closes it gently. Often reread, the dust jacket, a silhouette of the dark bird on a branch, has shifted and its colors are faded to near-gray.

She begins to remove the coarse, muslin-like bedspread, a near colorless shade like the sand dunes with just the slightest design of the yellow and green of the coastal buckwheat that grows out of them. The beige sham, by contrast, is sleek to touch, catching the light of the lamp beside her bed. She pulls it aside, and there, atop her pillow, in his familiar hand, is her name flowing in large script across his personal stationery.

"Ellie, Ellie," she cries. "He's written me something!" Her hand trembles as she tries to open it.

Ellie is at the door. "Let me..."

Ellie zips her finger under the flap. Shakily Suzan takes the letter and sits on the side of the bed. Ellie kneels in front of her. "Mom, everyone could tell how much he loved you..."

Suzan begins to read, but cannot manage. Ellie gently takes the letter from her hands, "Let me, Mom."

"Yes, Ellie read it to me."

> My dearest Suze, my lifelong love,
>
> I left you sleeping moments ago, darling. You were curled up, nearly on your stomach, your lovely breasts on display as if to call me back. In a moment, I will hear you stirring and bring

your first cup of coffee laced with cream. We'll begin another day. I hope mostly for another ordinary day, you accommodating my habits and me yours. But wait, my dearest. I've misspoken. No day is ordinary with you. Nor was last weekend at the symphony in S.F. an ordinary evening... and the Hyatt played its same magic on us.

The day is beautiful already, just the day for fishing in the cove once you're up and about. I lay awake during the night (a habit of old men like me) musing about you and me, how wonderful it has been, Suze, to be your husband. From the day we met on February 21, 1970, (Aren't I good?) I have known it could be this way, us at peace with ourselves and with the world. I would gladly pay the price of all that time again just to have you for this time. Was it Jacob who waited so long for Rachel? At least we've not had to deal with a trickster father.

Even when you resisted my efforts over the years while you were married to David, I prayed and hoped. When we lost track of each other, I always found you. Remember those times? During the lapses of time, you were never out of my mind. I'm reminiscing now.

Even after you left David, I nearly lost you. I remember agonizing in my letters. I still can hardly believe this kind of love exists. When you finally divorced David, you came to me. We met at Half Moon Bay. The next day, we went to the Hyatt in San Francisco, and I took you to the top of the Mark where we sat until the last seating. Several months later we went to Paris, and I prayed. Again I committed every part of my being, trying to trade promises with God. You were there with me on the Pont des Arts when I pledged to you any time remaining for us.

"Mom, you knew him all that time?" Ellie looks to her mother, pressing her hands against her knees, standing, holding the letter in the air. There's no accusation in her tone, just surprise. She kneels again, placing her hands on her Mother's knees, searching her face for her expression.

"Yes, Ellie. I've wanted to tell you our story. For my own selfish reasons, I need someone else on this earth to understand who I've lost, and what he meant to me."

Ellie continues reading, welling up,

> I think the most significant thing we have given ourselves is this well-earned haven. If ever I leave you, or rather, when I do, please live on here Suze, in Belle Haven as if I am still by your side. I will sell out my shares at Dairico and put the deed in your name. It will be completely yours, and then on to Ellie when your time comes. It's a graceful home and has taken on your elegance.

Suzan draws in her breath, caught short, thinking the house was owned between them. Ellie looks up, and then continues to read.

> But for now, at least temporarily, let's live a little larger. I've a plan to take you to Paris again. Will you go with me, my bride? This is your invitation, so hold on to it (although I won't change my mind).
>
> I want to see you there standing with me again on that narrow footbridge, gazing down at the Seine, so beautifully lighted, and flowing beneath. This time we shall thank the Almighty for this time we're having now, these ten years. I picture you there so often.
>
> Leaving you that morning back in '70 after our long night together on that plane, I hastened over to pray at Notre Dame, pleading that we could be together, that I could have two lives, as it were. I then went to the foot bridge, so popular to lovers for some reason, and I committed myself to God once again, promising anything to be with you. There in the mist of morning, it was not unlike the last moments at Orly when we parted. I'm often taken back to that moment, the mist surrounding you like a Madonna.

A SEASON OF MISTS

And so, as I said, I want to go a third time to say a prayer of gratitude. That very first time, alone, I cried there, not knowing if I would ever see you again. I was so torn. I went to Les Deux Magots, where Hemingway sometimes wrote, (not that he knew up from down about love) to write you that first letter. Everyone was going about his/her business, sitting outdoors having a café au lait, or a demitasse, while chatting or sipping silently alone.

My world had changed, and it seemed everything around me had been affected, colored over. The bells of St.-Germaine-des-Pres rang as I sat there outdoors under those large heaters. The table was hardly conducive to writing, but I was determined to write you. I found a post office and got back to Orly just in time to catch my plane to Buenos Aires. I wish we had those first letters.

You were so brave, darling, bringing your babies onboard that flight all alone. You looked so winsome, unaware of your beauty. You were so stern looking after I made that crack, I nearly laughed. I was so travel weary, having come from Kenya. I thought it was my misfortune to be seated in such close quarters with a young mother and two children. You warmed up to me when I helped with the children. After all, I have four of my own. I had seen it all before. It didn't faze you when Ellie threw up. Motherhood is something to admire in a woman, and I could see how intent you were to do it well. I, too, have experienced your good mothering. You're all woman, mi mujer.

I found myself falling for you. Then when I heard how you had helped the children out there on the desert, I fell hard. So rare is it, darling, to know someone who has that kind of compassion to endure the hardships you did. I believed you could change the world, light up your corner, so to speak. Gandhi said, "In a gentle way you can shape the world." You have that gentle way. Long into the flight when I first kissed you, you blushed. You heard my story about being a Jew in the Netherlands and escaping the times they caught me.

Sniffling, Ellie says, "Mom, the rest of the letter is for you, not me. In the morning, I want to hear the whole story. Try to sleep, Mom, we both need it."

The wave of family

Suzan sleeps long without waking, cushioned from the shock of Da's going by Ellie's love and understanding. Even so, the sun hasn't yet lit the ocean. She waits in bed until, swollen, it comes across the tall bluffs behind them.

She has begun to tell her story. Surely, Ellie will understand about the years she was growing up while her mother was alone. Suzan tends to lie near the middle where they slept, where the mattress has begun to give way. His side of the bed is left undisturbed. She stretches her hand under the covers across the bed to his side.

She rises and sees elusive patches of blue, broken clouds and the trailing vapors lifting, like the feeble smoke of a dying fire. She suddenly remembers he won't experience it. It is her and Da's kind of day. She returns to her pillow, face down, weeping into it. She doesn't know which is worse, the day brightly filled-in with color or a foggy day without escape.

The tri-folded letter on bond paper is close by. She will never stop reading it, and it will wear at the folds and around the edges over time. It will change in color, and one day Ellie will retrieve it from Suzan's belongings as a keepsake.

When she was just out of college, Da taught Ellie to cook omelets. "You need to learn from the best," he'd said. Now, she slips a yellow, steaming creation out of the skillet onto Suzan's plate. Suzan cuts into the omelet, and the gruyere cheese oozes and slides over the mushrooms.

"Half, Ellie, only half. Please. Sit down with me. I see you found the seedless raspberry jam in the pantry. Arthur orders that for us from the Trappist Monks."

Ellie had begun answering the phone yesterday, fielding those conveying condolences, responding to the family, and giving advice on where they might stay. Da's four children are coming.

"Their flights come into Portland early this morning, and they'll be here before lunch. They've found places to stay in the village. I'm glad it's off season." She tells Suzan now, glad she hadn't told her mother about their imminent arrival the evening before.

Although there is a trace of swelling in her face, to Ellie, she appears more rested, less dazed, more prepared to face family.

"I knew they were coming. Oh, Ellie, they're heartbroken, I know. Are the grandchildren coming along?"

"Just the little ones, Corrie and Dusty," Ellie says.

Of course, Casey, Daan and Charlotte are too busy. They're at that age, Suzan thinks. Maureen's Casey runs track, and nothing interferes with track. Daan and Charlotte must have extracurricular activities as well. As for the little ones, she's the only grandmother they've ever known.

Suzan applies her *Lancôme* foundation, hiding the circles beneath her eyes as best she can. She dresses as for a walk on the beach in something he has given her: a soft-pink sweatshirt, edged in satin. She might have picked her oldest dark sweatshirt, but she wants to appear as if she is coping. Ellie and she stay busy, preparing the house for company, planning menus. They carry in wood that Frank has split for the fireplace, and the fragrance of the freshly split wood perfumes the house.

By hand, Suzan launders her own tears out of the saffron robe that Ellie tried on. She hangs it in her bathroom, smiling again at the sight of Ellie. They've never had the same taste. At three, she refused to wear dresses, and they hung in her closet like doll clothes.

Late morning, his children converge. They've joined up, and only two rental cars pull in, their tires crunching on the stone drive. Suzan opens the double doors to the foyer. The air smells of the young pines Da and she have planted along the drive up the hill and mingles with the salt air. Paul, Phillip, Maureen and Mary come in behind the grandchildren. Dusty, belonging to Philip, swoops his thick, dark hair away from his forehead with a twist of his whole body.

At seven, a tender age, he embraces her quickly around her waist, his head flat against her stomach, "Grandma, don't cry."

But, silently she does as tears well up at the sight of them. She embraces tiny Cora, also belonging to Philip.

A SEASON OF MISTS

At four, Corrie lunges forward, hugging Suzan's neck as she stoops. Corrie's hands go to hold Suzan's face. "Are you sad, Grandma?"

The pink of her shirt is splotchy now, and Suzan sees the evidence of their sadness in their faces. Dusty distracts himself and steps over to examine a sculpted blue heron, smoothing his hand down the bronze neck. "He's standing on one leg," he says.

"That's to preserve his body heat," Phillip says.

Over his time there, Dusty will touch the several sculptures they've acquired. Indeed, though touching is discouraged, some are irresistible with a patina as seductive as satin. Suzan will let him experience the art in his own way. He will wander through the wide door into her studio and study a palette she has left beside an unfinished work. He will lift the dust cover over others. He will toy with a seashell from the crude shelf, built to hold paints and brushes.

Suzan looks up to the adults, squeezing Corrie around the waist. She's grown taller since summer. Her legs are long, and she reminds Suzan of a little filly. Suzan stands.

Da's children, so self-assured, seem to be coping well with their father's death. She grasps the hand of each, looks into their faces. The family greets Ellie from across the entrance. Ellie doesn't leave the open area of the kitchen. She pushes the still-warm, cinnamon-crusted muffins she has made to the center of the island and reaches for cups. "Welcome," she says.

The warm kitchen air is redolent of coffee and fresh muffins. What Ellie doesn't say in words, she often says in gestures. She continues her prep for lunch. She watches her mother speaking with Paul. His hand is on her shoulder.

The siblings compare their flights, congratulating themselves for having coordinated their arrivals into PDX. Everyone mills about for a bit, coffee cup in hand, looking for a chair or a window to look out toward the view of the ocean from this higher vantage point.

"Is that the cove?" Da's oldest son, Paul, asks, pointing to the smallest cove to the left of the footpath, directly below Belle Haven.

Nearly all gray at fifty-seven, Paul wears his hair much like his father did. It will also stay thick and turn a silvery white. His yellow polo shirt is taut against his wide chest. His tanned arms are covered with smooth dark hair. The breadth of his shoulders is greater than his father's. To Suzan, Paul's bearing exhibits strength and confidence. His voice is deeper and stronger than Da's and without the strong Dutch accent. Da's grandson Dusty hangs about Paul. Paul rubs his head and draws him close against his leg.

Da was proud of his oldest son's success. Suzan remembers him showing her his biography, proudly touting Paul's integrity and success as a businessman. Reading without pausing, Da had read:

> Paul Vandivere serves as the Chairman and Chief Executive Officer of Dairico Dairy Corp. He also serves as its President. It was he who founded the firm in 1973. He also co-founded and served as Chairman of the Board of Sunrise Organic Dairy. He serves as a Member of the Advisory Board of Chicago Investment Partners. Previously, he served as a Director of Sunrise Organic Holding Corp. Mr. Vandivere received a dual B.S. degree in Business and Engineering from the University of California at Berkeley.

Maureen and Mary come to the window behind Paul. Phillip, truly gifted but introverted when in the company of his brother, has pulled Dusty toward him. He holds back, his arms crossed around Dusty's chest. Dusty pulls away and turns to face his dad. Flipping his hair out of habit, Dusty says, "Did Grandpa die outside in the ocean?"

An enervating silence prevails.

As if cued, Suzan steps to the fore, facing away from them, looking toward the ocean scape, telling them what she witnessed the moments he was dying. She turns and puts her arm through Paul's. She is tenderer toward him, perhaps because he was born to Da when Da was only eighteen.

"The volunteer fire department came in less than five minutes, but he was gone. The paramedics tried to resuscitate him." She pauses to swallow, a catch in her throat. "He was happy here. He didn't think about death. He always anticipated the next day."

Mary, who rarely afforded to come for summer vacation, peers into the faces of the others, as if they should challenge Suzan. Behind Suzan's back, her head goes from one to the other.

She steps in front of Paul, her feet apart, saying, "He was so far away from us, clear out here. Why did he choose this place, so far away?"

Short and rotund, she lifts her arms, and lets them fall back to her side. "That path certainly doesn't look safe. It would be so easy to stumble. Are you sure he didn't fall?"

Mary now turns to Suzan, "I suppose he used those steps coming to and from the beach. Was he ever short of breath?"

Her always florid cheeks have turned an even darker pink. To Suzan she seems accusatory, her words salted with sarcasm.

"His asthma didn't bother him as much here." Somehow, in Mary's mind this must be Suzan's fault. Doesn't she believe how he died? Suzan wants to defend the steep steps down to the beach they had hired to be carved into the rocky slope, complete with a handrail they have had to replace every year, but she stops. She wants to point out the small landings with stumps where one can sit to rest on the way up, but she doesn't.

One by one, except for Paul, they turn away from the window. Ellie pours more coffee. After the heavy silence, the catching up with each other continues. Maureen says to Phillip, "I'm so glad you don't have to travel as much as Dad did with his job."

Phillip says, "Well, I'm not getting paid as well, either."

Paul remains in front of the window, his hands clasped behind his back. Phillip feels he has misstepped in the course of his career and wishes he were more senior. But he will always appear a tenderfoot. Prizes, such as there are in life, are hard to win and harder for some than others.

The first tense moments of receiving them over, Suzan feels she has safely sailed into harbor. Like tying herself to the dock, she brings out a coloring book for Corrie and seats her at the kitchen table. The big oak captain's chair corrals Corrie as she slides onto her knees and hunches over a scene of "The Three Little Pigs."

Suzan has framed one of her crayon-colored pictures from when she was here last and placed it in the hall half-bath. She'll show her in a minute. All the flowers are outlined in black, fiercely colored in with reds and yellows.

"What color are pigs, Grandma?" Leaning on her elbows, she holds up the box of sixty-four crayons with both hands. After turning her head, she says, "I want to color the ocean, just if Uncle Paul will get out of my way."

"Then you need different paper. Come over here to Grandpa's desk where you can see the ocean better."

Suzan pulls out Da's chair and opens the writing table, exposing his fountain pen and the bottle of black ink. Her heart constricts. There, too, is the engraved silver letter opener she gave him for their anniversary, inscribed: *Three decades, with love, Suze;*. She tucks it into a drawer. Da and she had acted as if this day would never come when others would look at their most personal things.

Phillip loves to write privately both prose and poetry and steps over to handle the pen. He lifts the square bottle of ink, and then explores how to load the gold Waterman, lifting the plunger. Suzan can see that he covets it.

As he fiddles, one bulbous drop falls like blood onto the ecru stationery. Suddenly, Suzan remembers with a smidgen of joy that Da had shed no blood. He had died, his body unscathed. But earlier losses come to mind, like heavy, unwanted clumps of seaweed dragged in out of the ocean on one's fishing line. Matthew's violent death is suddenly fresh. Recalling the baby she didn't bear, the hint of joy is quickly overcome. She blots the ink. There are few. Da was always careful.

From her studio, she brings a fresh piece of sketching paper for Corrie. Phillip closes the pen, placing it where he found it. "Here Cor, I need one of your hugs," he says to Corrie huskily. She stands on the chair and complies. Phillip felt strongly connected with his father, both loving to write their thoughts.

A child's comfort cuts through to the heart, and Phillip holds her as memories of his father's prolific letters course through his mind.

"Why didn't Mommy come?" she says.

"They needed her at the hospital." He speaks of Michelle, his wife, a nurse practitioner. Phillip depends on her when decisions are to be made, and he misses her.

The burial place

Suzan wears the ring she instinctively took from Da's finger after she followed his body behind the ambulance. Too big, it twists on her finger. It is set with three diamonds, one for each decade. She told him when she had it designed. It too is inscribed and says: *love for three decades, Suze*. It belongs back on his hand, she thinks. Why has she credited their love with three decades when only a few years were theirs to claim?

Not this telling ring, she thinks, but some of his personal things can go to them, if they ask. She can see that Phillip would treasure the antique fountain pen. After Mary expressed her doubts, Suzan's capacity for compassion was blocked temporarily. Now, she feels tender toward Da's children, acknowledging their loss. She feels less defensive. Maybe she'll ask them if they'd like something personal of his.

"We should talk about the arrangements," Paul says, still looking out the window, his back toward the others.

"What's been done so far?" He turns to Suzan. "I forgot to mention, Teri is here. She stayed back in the room to catch up a bit from the night flight. Coming from Denver was quite a trek. In order to get here this morning, we had to fly into Seattle then hop down to Portland. Otherwise, we would have been delayed a day. I'll run get her after lunch. We made arrangements as soon as we could after you called from the hospital."

"I understand. It will be so good to see Teri," Suzan says. "As to the planning, I've asked the local mortician about cremation after a family viewing. The memorial service would be the day following the cremation."

Mary reacts with a sudden turn toward Suzan. "But who…?"

Suzan continues, "I thought we would let go his ashes into the ocean, maybe spread them from Frank's charter boat. Frank's a good friend. Your dad really enjoyed going out deep sea fishing with him. Your dad became like part of the crew."

Mary is forty-eight and single, a nun. "But it's against our beliefs," she says, again looking toward the others to support her. Her entire face is suddenly more ruddy. Her hands go to her hips.

Maureen, two years younger than Mary, says quietly, "No need to get into a tiff, Mary. I just thought we would do a graveside service when we bury him alongside Mother."

In her job as a software engineer, she competes well. She makes a strong case for women's equal standing in careers that have been the stronghold of men.

Very trim, she's wearing a flattering wool sweater set and pants of the same dye lot, probably by Eileen Fisher, a new designer. The blue matches her milky blue eyes. Her hair is lightened and highlighted, cut with a very straight edge, so that it swings forward into her face as she leans toward Mary to make her point.

"In Maryland?" Phillip, the youngest, asks thinking of the expense. "That's a long way to ship his body. We'd all have to fly back there, and I don't have room for everyone at my place. Also, Michelle is still working the night shift."

Corrie interrupts. "Grandma, the ocean isn't the same blue as the sky."

Ellie goes to Corrie in her mother's stead and pulls out all the blues and blue-greens, suggesting she mix them. Corrie has colored in the sky on the top quarter of the page. Not a very big sky. She has left room for a very big ocean. "Your horizon is nicely done," Ellie says.

"I want Grandma to see," Corrie says.

"Remember to notice where the light is coming from," Suzan says over her shoulder, turning back to the family.

"But Grandma, it comes from the sun."

Suzan shrinks at the idea of Da being taken to Maryland. Why hadn't she asked him? If that's the case, she'll not go. There they stand, his children, she thinks, all intact, not knowing their father had loved her for three decades, not knowing how her heart wants to be with his very body.

"I'd rather he be here, either buried or cremated, preferably cremated." Suzan states her position one more time.

A SEASON OF MISTS

Mary, who lives in rural Massachusetts, says, "Far better in Maryland than all the way out here in Oregon. I agree with Maureen. Alongside Mother is the best place. His plot is already there. Even his name and date of birth are on it." She fiddles with the knot of drab brown hair on top her head.

Suzan thinks, *Oregon is not a foreign country*, but says, "I'll make the call to the mortuary, if that's what we all agree to do."

The siblings are silent, not expecting her to comply so readily. Paul, then Phillip nod in agreement. Paul says, "I'll make the calls to Maryland this morning before it gets too late."

Ellie looks from the kitchen, regretting her mother's agreement with Mary and Maureen. It seems as if her mother should have the say. If Ellie and Mary were sisters, they would be enemies, polar opposites. Even the way Mary dresses, like the nun she is, skirt mid-calf, an ugly brown, annoys Ellie. She probably never exercises and looks frumpy and much older than Ellie's mother. There are several rolls of fat bulging through her blouse. Her poorly supported, large breasts are slack and have pitched down as if toward the children she bends over as she teaches. It is known that she sings in a choir, and Ellie imagines she dominates the sopranos. Ellie rather likes Maureen, seemingly imperturbable with a polished protective veneer, her emotions in check; she doesn't go on about things. Ellie feels a twinge of guilt for her thoughts and preemptive judgment of Mary.

Corrie is coloring in a very rough ocean, especially as it rushes into the coves, where she has tried to color white over the blue water and black for the rocks being washed over by a wave. A figure represents her deceased grandfather fishing, and she adds a rather large looking silvery fish to the end of his line.

Belle haven

Ellie's mean thoughts about Mary are interrupted by the phone. It's Madeleine, Ellie's friend in San Francisco. Ellie takes the call in the guestroom, and Suzan hangs up the receiver, turning back to the family. All she heard Madeleine say was, "Are you managing? I know it's tough." Ellie returns fifteen minutes later.

After lunch, a quick chili, Maureen and Phillip help in the kitchen. The others find comfortable chairs. Dusty is bored. After his calls to Maryland, Paul asks his nephew if he'd like a walk. Dusty says, "Down to the cove where Grandpa drowned?"

Paul puts down the *New Yorker* he's reading, rubs the head of his look-alike nephew and says, "He didn't drown, Dustin. His heart stopped."

"What makes a heart stop?"

Phillip calls, "Be careful son, and do as your uncle says."

Maureen, who shares Ellie's habit of riding a bicycle, is somewhat curious about Ellie and asks, "Have you always lived on the west coast?"

"No, I grew up in California, then at sixteen we moved to North Virginia," she says, dumping the small amount of guacamole left over into the trash, double wrapping the remaining chips because of the damp air. "Mother had taken a job as a civil servant for the Air Force satellite tracking station in Sunnyvale, California, and they transferred her to work at Vandenburg Air Force Base as a writer. That was in 1985."

"Now that you're in San Francisco, is it hard to bike in the city?"

"My favorite place to bike now is near the Presidio. There's a large bike network and a coalition in the city. They've made good progress." The muscles in her shoulders and arms are apparent through her simple tee-shirt.

A SEASON OF MISTS

Her response seems to make Maureen go quiet, as if they have nothing else in common. Da's children understand they know very little about Ellie, even though she makes them welcome and caters to them. They only see her on summer holidays. They have spoken together about how private a person she is. They concluded she is too private to know. They're right. Few people know Ellie as well as she knows herself. Her expressions are warm but guarded.

Suzan always wanted everyone to come at once, and every year they planned for the next. Still, Suzan and Ellie felt separate from the rest, except Teri, who chats with them readily in the kitchen or on beach walks. Ellie always took the only other suite in the house. Belle Haven was the hub, and families wandered up and down during the day, enjoying the beach. The cottages in which they stayed were not elegant, the kitchens small and the furniture sparse. Da was their center.

Maureen doesn't take the conversation any further. She picks up this week's *New Yorker*, looking at the cover of the cartoonish contestants for Miss America.

Ellie knows she'll never really be considered part of Da's family. She's moved closer to her mother now to the west coast, to San Francisco, a different, more tolerant world than theirs, one they wouldn't likely understand.

Mary drives to the village to pick up Teri. They return, and Teri is shown the cove. She moves more closely to Maureen and Mary and takes their hands.

Teri is petite, with short, dark hair, wispy around her neck and cheeks and has shining brown eyes. To mother is her nature, and she'll be doing stand-in mothering for Philip's children, Corrie and Dusty, through the afternoon, unable to detach herself from their playful moments. Likely, she will take them to search the beach for shells and sea glass.

She loves the village even during tourist season, finding a piece of sculpture reminiscent of Rodin perhaps for her garden or a bear carving by the Inuit in Alaska. She always goes to see Suzan's paintings in Samantha's By the Sea gallery and insists on paying full price for those she chooses.

Paul is still at the cove with Dusty. They have climbed above the cove and are standing on a large, jagged rock, an impermeable black rock that looks like a puzzle piece that would fit in the hallowed space below where Da died. In what century did a tide lift that rock, creating the ledge where passersby can stand to watch the sea change and swirl in rotations? He has seen a painting by Suzan of this scene, the only one of hers that hangs in the house. Otherwise, her paintings of the past have been sent to the gallery, where she has developed a reputation for seascapes.

Teri says to no one in particular, "I wish Charlotte and Daan were here. They both had SAT exams to take. Why didn't Casey come?" She pauses. "Things will never be the same without Dad."

She turns from the window to find Suzan. "And you, Suzan, are you truly okay? I don't know how you hold up, especially with a house full of us. This is such a shock. It was just a week ago when you two stopped over in Denver after you returned from Geneva."

Reminded of their last trip, how they relived the long-ago imagined visit to Geneva spoken of in one of his old letters to her, Suzan can't continue the conversation and diverts Teri's attention. She feels her face twitch as if she's developed a tic.

"Come see Corrie's picture. Grandpa caught a fish. Wouldn't he have been happy?" She says.

Returning, Paul encircles Teri with his arms. A quiet pause lingers between them. With his arm around her shoulder, Paul reports that the mortuary they've chosen will meet the airplane, finish preparing Da's body for the family viewing and arrange the service. The children agree to buy the coffin Suzan had selected, even though she had only rented it for the viewing. Mary will submit an obituary to the *Washington Post*. They arrange their flights into Dulles for tomorrow. They arrange for the body to be on the same plane. Making reservations ahead, Paul and Teri will stay at the Willard, downtown D.C. The burial will be in Maryland beside their mother early next week.

Later, in the afternoon, Paul and Phillip walk beneath the extended porch, looking at the supporting timbers, pulling on a bit of draping wiring from the furnace. Paul measures with his hands the thickness of the retainer wall, remarking on the solid rock behind it. They look at the caulked seals around the doors and windows. "It's well maintained," says Phillip. "What's your guess on its worth?"

"No idea. The deed is in Dairico's name. The will gives her everything except what's invested in Dairico. She'll have to take what money she gets and live someplace else. She'll be a wealthy woman, but she won't have Belle Haven. It will remain titled to Dairico."

"Is that what Dad wanted... for her to leave? We should know that first." Philip says. Phillip envies his brother's thriving industry, but especially he envies that his father had become an investor in his brother's business. *Was Paul favored?* He wonders.

"The will, and that's what counts, doesn't mention Belle Haven going to her, only the money he left invested with Morgan Stanley. Dairico actually purchased the house. The money came from his earnings at the business, but the shares don't go to her. This can become the most expensive and well-appointed weekly rental in the village. If we hold on to it, it will only gain in value."

Suzan and Ellie are on the porch out of earshot, talking quietly. They descend the rocky, gouged-out steps toward the beach and walk to the village, giving Da's children time to settle the interment details among themselves.

Maureen and Mary stand talking in the kitchen. They pull out drawers and look beneath the sink as if they had never really examined the house before. They appear to be looking at it as potential owners.

"These oak cabinets are beautifully crafted. The carpenter must have been someone local," Maureen says quietly, rubbing the granite counter lengthways following its veins of beige and black.

"The stove is a Viking. The kitchen is all custom-built. They've put a lot of thought into the whole house. It's a lot of space for two people. You have to admire her taste," Maureen continues.

"Only the best," Mary says. "He spoiled her." She doodles her initials with one of her father's finely sharpened pencils left near the phone, testing the unused pink eraser after she draws a group of attached triangles. Smudged on one side, she replaces it in the blue ceramic pen holder.

"Well, he was also very particular in everything he set out to do," Maureen says.

Teri has taken Corrie with the buckets and shovels to the beach. The tide is far out, and the revealed shells look like sequins, winking in the sun. Corrie is hardly recognizable, she is so bundled up. An adult size scarf comes unlooped when she bends to dig. Determined, she slings it back and fills the buckets over and over. They're sandy, wet and cold when they return.

After a warm bath, Corrie curls up with Teri in Da's leather chair with something out of the children's section. She listens closely to *The Star-bellied*

Sneeches. She asked why some were star-bellied and others not. No one but Dr. Seuss really knows. She falls asleep during the answer. Teri moves carefully out of the chair and covers her with a cashmere afghan the color of Corrie's hair: soft beige, with wheat-like streaks.

Later, as Ellie prepares the broth, Teri cleans the clams Phillip and Dusty have gone out for. Phillip makes a run to Rosie's before closing time for French bread.

"Pick up a chocolate cream pie, too, in case someone wants dessert," Teri says.

"I do, I do!" Dusty says.

When Phillip returns, Suzan suggests they may want something of their father's. Phillip asks for Da's fountain pen, Maureen asks for the shaving mug. Paul doesn't ask for anything, but accepts Da's college ring when Suzan offers it. No one asks about the Rolex. It's still at the mortuary, and Suzan has forgotten about it. Maureen goes through his ties, sorting by color and style for her husband Bill. Such pride Suzan had taken buying them before they married when he wore one every day. Remembering his signature omelets, Mary wants the omelet pan. Would Suzan mind?

None of the furniture belonged in the siblings' first home, and Da's children have no attachment to the sculptures or the variety of paintings and prints from museums around the world. Representing the god of agriculture, the black Chiwara by the Bambara of Mali is featured against an oak shelf.

Maureen wants the fishing gear for her son, Casey, and sorts through it in the garage. Suzan helps her break down the poles and put them into their green leather cases. The unwieldy tackle box is emptied into a small cardboard box. Suzan layers the tackle into it with plastic bags and wax paper. "He'll have to pick out another tackle box," she says. "Let me know, and we... I'll get it for him."

After the clams and many compliments to Ellie, she finishes preparing the salmon and potatoes au gratin for dinner. Teri makes the salad, following Ellie's instructions, slicing kiwi and strawberries over butter lettuce, mixing the raspberry vinaigrette and adding a little crème fraiche to toss it just before they serve. Paul makes a fire with freshly split cedar logs, wet but dry at the core causing the crackling fire to hiss and sizzle.

Corrie sleeps on and looks so comfortable no one has the heart to waken her. Suzan touches her slight shoulder. "Time for dinner."

Corrie wakens, and for a moment looks puzzled. She clambers to sit between Suzan and Teri. Dusty is sitting tall next to his uncle Paul.

Suzan, looking down to the end of the table at Paul where Da should be sitting, lifts a Waterford champagne glass filled with the champagne she has poured all around. "He would have wanted us to celebrate his love for life," she says.

"Hear, hear," they say.

"Without Dad, I could never have developed the career as a statistician that I have, nor could I have understood all the ins and outs of the culture at the World Bank. It was an elderly colleague of Dad's who attended that original conference in Bretton Woods after WWII who supported my being hired by the World Bank, but I was so green. Only Dad could have taught me the ropes. He encouraged me to stay with it." His voice falters, "He was a good old dad." Phillip's voice doesn't have the same timbre as Paul's, and he sounds younger than his forty-five years.

"Hear, hear," they say.

Maureen picks up her glass. Her hand shakes, and the champagne laps the crystal and makes tiny waves.

"Casey probably wouldn't be with us had Mom and Dad not found and paid for the best pediatric heart surgeon in the world. And now he runs track." She wants to say more, but her voice chokes. They raise their glasses.

Mary, by now, feels the effect of the champagne. Her round cheeks are nearly scarlet. She's ready to speak before Maureen has finished. There's urgency in her voice. "Because of Dad's encouragement, I've devoted my whole life to service to Christ…"

"Hear, hear," they say before she can go on.

Paul speaks as last of the children. As CEO of Dairico, and the various other positions he holds, he is accustomed to speaking extemporaneously. Usually a person of few words, Paul speaks in an uncharacteristically halting manner.

"Dad bought me my first Holstein heifer calf. We picked it out together, and I joined the Potomac 4-H. Dad became a pack leader and went to nearly all the shows in which our group competed. We always took first prizes…

remember all those championship purple ribbons that hung in my room? I owe my first interest in going into the dairy business to Dad."

As the oldest, Paul seems to be assuming his place as patriarch of the family. Perhaps, it is owing to his wealth and his confident manner, but the others seem respectful and accepting. It seems natural that he has taken the end chair at the table. It had seemed natural that he made the calls to Maryland and negotiated with Suzan.

"He taught me to dig for clams. He showed me how to watch for those little breathing holes in the sand when the tide was out." Dusty lifts his glass of milk.

Ellie toasts Da, saying, "He was a friend to me." She might have said, "He made my mother very happy."

Corries says, "He bounced me on his knees."

As she picks up her glass, it tips and the milk spills.

"What would it be like to have a meal without spilled milk?" Phillip says, getting up to sop it up. Corrie tries to help with her napkin. Her father settles her back into her chair.

"Sitting still would be the most help."

Phillip is embarrassed that Corrie even tried to give a toast.

Teri quotes a poem her father-in-law had written about the grandchildren, rhyming their names, capturing their endearing qualities.

They find other reasons, like the frequency of their father's letters, to raise their glasses, until they fall silent. Subdued, the conversation picks up when the food is passed, but the general tone is somber. Suzan removes the champagne glasses especially designed for the centennial and pours the French Sauvignon Blanc, one Da had selected. She serves the potatoes from where she sits, first to Corrie, so her portion can cool.

Later that evening, Teri takes Suzan down to the mortuary for a last visit with Da's body. Ellie stays back. The room is dim, but the open coffin seems to have a light trained on it. Suzan reaches in and straightens his pink and grey tie. She is having difficulty breathing. Her hands shaking, she removes the diamond-set gold ring from her finger and pushes it over the cold, stiff knuckle, wanting it to go with him to the grave. She'll mention it to Paul before they go. She shudders. She pats his bit of a paunch, but unexpectedly, it isn't soft. Repelled by the rigidity, she sucks in her breath, stifling her sob.

A SEASON OF MISTS

Teri puts her arm around Suzan's waist. Suzan responds, and they quietly stand, linked arm and arm before the coffin, away from the infusion of light.

The whole family sits around the fire through the evening, reminiscing. The cedar logs burn hot and quickly, and Paul adds a large chunk of seasoned fir to settle it. Beneath it the fire is soothed to a steady orange bed of glowing embers. They tell stories of their childhood. They laugh and cry. They tell stories on each other. Suzan carries the sleeping Corrie away from the hearth.

"You always were his favorite." Suzan hears someone say.

"I don't remember that part," comes the answer.

The log slips, and the fire spits new flames, crackling and popping as it buckles and resettles. The embers ascend and are quickly extinguished as they rise.

"Remember how Mother and Dad were naturalized as citizens the very day Hawaii became a state in 1958? Phillip, you were too young. What were you, three?"

Phillip sits at the piano, looking through the sheet music. "Play something, Phil," Maureen says.

Turning on the bench to face them, Phillip changes the subject abruptly and says "No", not wanting be the one without the memory so accessible to the others.

"I do remember being in Kenya on that huge tea plantation, the American school we attended and those scratchy wool uniforms in the winter."

He swivels and puts the music away, closes the piano and leans into it, his arms around his head. He is fixed with his face buried, and they see his back heaving as he sobs. Paul swivels his chair away. He looks into the fire and rubs his forehead so as not to allow the loss they share to overcome him.

It will be an early morning get-up. Other than the place of burial, they have had no disagreements. Suzan has heard the quaver in Phillip's voice. She leaves them still talking in the library at near midnight.

Corrie is sleeping over, and Suzan has opened Da's side of the bed for her. She sleeps in one of Suzan's tee-shirts, and it has slipped over her pale slender shoulder. *An angel sleeps in his place,* she thinks.

The colors of an angry ocean

The bustle in the morning to sort out tickets and times of departure preclude any lengthy conversation before breakfast. When they arrive to say goodbye, they seem talked out from the night before, and quietly gather to watch the ocean from the glass porch, waiting for Ellie's call to breakfast. Someone says, "We should have a picture of the cove."

"I'll go down," Phillip says. His camera is very sophisticated. He returns with it from the car and switches the lens.

"Can we have pancakes? I can help. I use to help Grandpa crack the eggs." Dusty says.

Ellie is frying bacon. "You read my mind," she says.

Suzan finds a fresh cloth and napkins. Maureen and Mary set the table. Maureen goes behind Mary and straightens what she does. She refolds the napkins. Dustin attempts to make a pancake, and the batter drips across the griddle making a path of miniature lopsided circles that brown unevenly.

When Phillip returns, Ellie cooks each order separately, tucking the crisped bacon alongside. Corrie's are small but stacked three deep. She tucks in. Allowed to pour her own syrup, she smothers the cakes and floods the bacon.

When it's time for departure, the family is quiet again, perhaps an effort to extend the moments when they are together. Suzan feels included. She doesn't busy herself cleaning up. Ellie sits down and has her portion. Suzan aches for his family to become Ellie's and hers.

Finally, Paul takes a deep breath, "Thank you, Suzan, for receiving all of us at once, and thank you Ellie for the delicious food. I'm afraid it's time to go…"

Corrie's picture of an angry ocean is on the refrigerator. As well it might have been, she believes the tumultuous ocean to be the culprit in losing her grandpa. She, too, grieves. She stands beside the stick figure representing her grandfather and says, "It was a big wave, like this one."

The wave towers over her grandfather, and indeed its force would have pulled him into its eddy as it swirled around the cove. She crosses her arms and leans against the refrigerator, burying her face. Teri gently pulls her away.

"Please come for your holidays, Dusty, we'll go to the largest sea lion cave in the world, just south of here in Florence." Suzan says as the car doors slam.

"Me too!" Corrie says.

Corrie and Dusty want to ride with Teri and Paul, and they make the switch.

Da's body goes away as do his children. Suzan knows there probably won't be much contact with them until they review the will together. Until his last letter, she believed he had made certain the deed to Belle Haven was sorted out. *Without Belle Haven, without Da, this blended family probably won't be as close,* she thinks. No one could have left that large a legacy.

A strong surge of the grief, unfinished and interrupted, creeps like sludge into her gut as the family drives off. The weight of her sorrow is too great to contain. Nauseous, trembling, she turns for Ellie. Ellie removes her apron before she embraces her. They move inside, Suzan to the glassed porch. The fog drifts south, uncovering the colors most common in her art. She wishes for an overcast, dark day, even drizzling rain, to close out some of the possibilities of how to use this day. Ellie moves the *Oregonian* and sits on the coffee table in front of her mother. She blots the tears with a tissue.

"What, Mom? What?"

Suzan shrugs and wipes her eyes.

"Can we go to the gallery this afternoon?" Ellie leans her elbows on her knees and cups her face between her hands as if she's thinking through a problem.

"Why are you painting a wren somewhere in each picture? It's almost become part of your signature."

"Oh Ellie, I used to tell him he was like a wren, the 'King of the Fence' with his continued mating calls."

A pebble in the pocket

It's Ellie's last day, and they walk on the beach past the large pillar of stacked rock toward the village. Suzan speaks into the wind, which nearly swallows her words, "I have more to tell you about the years before Da and I married. I wasn't alone all that time. I had Da."

Ellie leans into her ear, "You've got to tell me everything."

Arriving at Rosie's they have strong, dark coffee and share a large cinnamon bun. The white icing has drizzled over the sides and crusted.

Suzan stirs the cream into her coffee slowly and says, "First, tell me about Madeleine. Even though you're sad about Da, you seem lighter hearted than when you were here in the summer. You're a little thin. You must be exercising your heart out."

Rosie brings a refill. She places a hand on Suzan's shoulder but says nothing. Suzan continues to stir the cream into her coffee, and then holds the mug with both hands, leaning her elbows on the wooden table, waiting.

"Mom, Maddy and I love each other, and we're going to be a family," Ellie says, not pausing as she traces the grooves in the scarred table with her index finger.

"We connected last spring through an off-site board meeting. Since then, we've planned our time around each other."

Separating the cinnamon roll with her slim fingers, she clears her throat and swallows. She doesn't allow time for her mother's reaction. Her sentences run together.

"We've applied to adopt a baby whose parents are dying of AIDS. We've been accepted, but he won't be available for another month. He had some health issues with his lungs initially. He was born prematurely. We've found a three bedroom and are moving in on the fifteenth of next month. We've named him Matthew after Matt. Right now, we're trying to be at the hospital for his feedings as often as we can. They're predicting he'll be three months when we bring him home. In our new place, there'll be a room for you too when you come."

"Ellie, I'm so glad you're telling me, but it's so much to absorb at one time... you with Madeleine and then a baby." She sets her cup down and reaches toward Ellie, leaving her arm resting on the table, her hand extended, her fingers open.

Suzan isn't surprised by Ellie's choice of Maddy. But she is overwhelmed just the same that Ellie is finally open and they can talk about her sexuality, even plan around it.

She only hopes Maddy is made of the same mettle. There will be a grandchild. Ellie and Maddy will make a home. *As strong and self-reliant as she thinks she is, Ellie needs this,* Suzan thinks. She needs to be anchored in family and the responsibilities and trust that come with being a partner. She needs to have this kind of love and companionship. She has postponed her own happiness too long. Rosie quietly pours more coffee and removes the empty plate and silverware. Before Suzan reaches for the cream, she extends her hand again and Ellie takes it.

"Ellie, when can I meet Madeleine?"

"As soon as possible. I haven't told Dad. I just can't, Mom. When we get little Matthew, he won't have a grandfather. If Da were only here…"

"Your father would have a hard time accepting a child who he would think is tainted by the evil of this world. He views HIV-AIDS as a Biblical plague. Let alone, sweetheart, what he would say about your caring for Madeleine."

"He'll never know about Maddy and me. I promise you that. Better yet, I've promised myself. But, we have so little contact, it won't be hard.

"But, Mom, what is this about you and Da knowing each other for so long?"

"I'll try to tell you the story. We waited many years. After Cora died in '89, we waited another year to marry. Even then, his children felt it was too soon. We had already leased this home together. It was only natural to buy it and come here. It was like the breaking up of the morning clouds for us to have a married life together."

"You've had Belle Haven all these years? I knew your paintings went back in time, but I didn't know the house was yours all along. No wonder it reflects your taste and feels like home," she laughs.

"I think it will be my mainstay, Ellie, I really do, if I can keep it. Belle Haven and you."

As they retrace their steps, the wind to their backs ruffling their jackets, Ellie reaches down for a small, wet, black, stone. Inside her pocket, she rubs it, and it's smooth against her thumb, polished by being cast by the sea to the shore over and over.

Mother is not surprised about Maddy, Ellie thinks. Neither is she surprised her mother had a lover those years after divorcing Dad. She hadn't known that Da and her mother had loved each other and were communicating long before they began having physical relations. Ellie is touched and happy for her mother having had a friend and lover over that hard period as a single, unsupported mom.

Their home in Santa Cruz over some of those years, which was just steps from the warm, approachable ocean, was idyllic and gilded in Ellie's memory. Then at puberty she became so confused. Then the move to the Vandenburg AFB and Matthew being killed. Those were hard years and deepened her tendency to quietly reflect.

They can see Belle Haven, and it's like a beacon to Ellie's soul. How wonderful if her mother could stay on as Da wished. She follows a wave out and walks quickly backward as another wave washes in, slithering under her feet before she knows it. She holds her sandals behind her back. The shiny sand of low tide is hard, and bubbles appear on its surface, break and disappear. Her mother wants to talk; her silent, reflective, self-contained mother is taking her into her confidence. Ellie wants to talk as well. New and old boundaries are being carefully stepped over, and they're coming in to a new kind of intimacy.

Ellie is discerning and has often longed to share confidences with her mother, the significant, consequential matters and the ragged edges of the heart, but all along, she thought it would be hard for her mother to think of her as a lesbian. With Matthew gone, she knows not having a biological grandchild will disappoint. But maybe Maddy's and her baby will win her over. Most children do. Maybe they'll be a family.

A SEASON OF MISTS

Ellie has ached for family. A door of communication is opening. Together, they're removing the debris, unjamming and opening it. They are both ready to understand and be forgiven for the secrets they've kept from each other.

When Matt died, Ellie's mother had grown unfamiliarly quiet for at least a year. Ellie had never felt so alone. In this moment, Ellie's residual anger toward the misguided driver who killed Matt is rekindled.

There is no one else except herself upon whom to count. Hopes for a family of his were struck down in that moment. She's it. Matt had held the strings to his mother's heart. He had always brought the sweetest girls home to meet her. Although it doesn't appear her mother will ever be dependent, Ellie wishes Matt were here to share her growing sense of responsibility for her emotionally. Matt would be thirty-four.

As a child, Ellie modelled her mother, the exterior shell of her: the discipline, the self-confidence, certainly her independence after the divorce, her stoicism after the death. She doesn't know it now, but she will emulate Suzan all the more with Maddy in her life. She'll be building in more structure with the purpose of making a home. Suzan always made a dependable, welcoming home for Matt and her, and Ellie wants to do as much for her new family.

Rubbing the pebble as they walk, Ellie works a plan. She'll extend for a week, and invite Maddy to come here to Belle Haven. This seems like the time for them to meet. Maddy can take a day to drive through the redwoods then follow along coastal Highway 101 on the next day. Ellie continues to plan. She wants Maddy to know her history, and that includes her mother's story. Also, she believes Maddy will be well received by her mother. If Maddy comes, Ellie thinks by extending her stay, she'll have more time to raise questions and get more information about the past.

By the time Suzan married Da, Ellie had her own apartment, but her mother remained her anchor. She hadn't understood the decision to marry the unknown Da and hadn't anticipated being introduced to a stepfather much older than her mother, a man nearly her grandmother's age when she passed. She hadn't expected her mother to leave California. She felt a bit abandoned. Maybe a lot.

Ellie fell hard for Da. How much he was like her grandfather Pop. She felt instantly welcomed. She came often especially in the summer and always left with the sense of longing to come back. She also fell in love with Belle

Haven and saw how content her mother had become. She transferred to a new branch in San Francisco.

"Mom, I'd like to stay on and have Maddy come up and meet you."

"Ellie, if she's part of you, I'd welcome her."

Suzan doesn't feel ready for life to move on. She wants more time to absorb her loss of Da. But Ellie's right. It's a good time to meet Maddy, before they move in together, before they get the baby. Ready or not.

Just below the path up to Belle Haven, like a call to prayer, Suzan hears the chords of the set of hand-tuned copper chimes she released to the breeze this morning. Sometimes when she had seen him coming up the path, she would untie a set briefly, to let him know she saw him coming. They were too noisy and repetitive otherwise, and sometimes they tangled in the wind. Ahead of Ellie as they climb, Suzan holds a kind of ritual for Da in her mind. She hears the caw, caw, caw of a strutting crow. She sees and feels the thrust of a seagull's wings to her right.

Perhaps their silent bald eagle will sit like a sentinel on the highest fir on the slope this evening. These comforting and familiar experiences, as she reaches for strength and acknowledges a higher power, will come, whether she paints, reads, stands waiting for the sun to shine through the skylights and the great windows, or as she bathes in her glassed bathroom exposed to the earliest light of the morning. Such vivid recall she has of him alive. Less and less she recalls the coffin or the cove.

Over time, she'll hold a series of mini-services as memories overtake her, unaware from where they spring, whether from a sight, a sound, a smell, the touch of silk or the rough tweed of a sofa pillow. Inevitably, she will turn toward him during the night. She will turn to lie flat on her back in those moments and talk to him in a whisper. The tears will slide down each side of her face and be absorbed by her pillow. She'll not regret their choices over the years. She'll keep a journal as if talking to him at the end of the day.

His memorial service in Maryland is not for her. Suddenly, now, she sees him coming down the steps to meet her, and she's glad Ellie can't see her face as she cries in disappointment.

She'll be alone climbing this path when Ellie leaves. She can't think of Ellie going. There is too much to be said in this place and at this time. How will it be between them when Maddy comes? She feels unprepared, but she feels hopeful. Ellie radiates an inner sureness. There will be a child in all his uniqueness to love and nurture. Suzan is tender toward him already because he's essentially parentless and came too soon into this world.

Ellie calls San Francisco, and Maddy is available for several days and will leave the next morning, Saturday, to arrive mid-day Sunday. *Suzan will be reassured when she meets and knows Maddy,* Ellie thinks. Ellie believes with her professional insights Maddy can help Suzan begin to heal emotionally.

The timing, telling her mother of Maddy, having her come, seems perfect. Ellie needs Maddy with her on this uncharted path forward in her relationship with her mother. There are many long-held confidences on each side, including her own history, while coming to accept her sexuality. Ellie has only ever loved another woman.

With Ellie and Maddy and baby Matthew together, Suzan will eventually become the matriarch of a new family. At the top of the steps, she looks back to Ellie and holds her hand out for the last few steps. They are breathless, drawing in great breaths, as they embrace.

Glowing primly, the sun slips into the horizon. It is the color of a ripening persimmon and lights up the clouds clustered before it. During the changing light, from the lustrous semi-darkness to dark, Ellie and Suzan talk. They forget about making supper. On into the darkness of that fall night they talk and listen, their softened voices are like the sh-sh-shush of the sibilant breaths of the ocean below them. They won't stir until well after midnight. It is Suzan who speaks to her regrets.

"I knew how you were struggling," Suzan says. "I know I seemed far away when we lost Matthew. I should have sought advice about how to help you. But now, Ellie, you seem settled and you remind me more of yourself as a girl. I couldn't confide in you otherwise."

"Mom, I couldn't tell when you were struggling. You didn't let on, and I was too caught up in my own confusion. I wanted so much to be a boy."

"I often wrote my heart to Da… but I never told anyone of the tendencies I saw in you. I didn't want to accept it. I was afraid for you, knowing how intolerant and cruel people can be. I know now how much you loved Sonja."

"I didn't think I could ever love anyone else. Matthew tried to introduce his friends, but all I could think of was Sonja.

"Mom, why couldn't you have let go of Da and just dated?"

"I didn't ever experience again what I had experienced with him. He had an exotic magnetism only I can understand. Some of that was the distance and separation, I'm sure. I suppose I was insecure and afraid, Ellie. Being pursued by him was the most affirming thing that ever happened to me. His words were the most intimate I'd ever heard. He introduced me to a whole new world, a world in which I wanted to belong. For me, it was even a different level of sophistication for which I was looking.

"Somewhere in my mind, I associated my own success with loving him. I have never laid it all out to anyone else. His pursuit of me and my being able to talk through letters, that and that he found me sexually appealing… the years just went by. I was working hard. I had blinders on. I can't answer your question, Ellie, but I believed in love. I do, I believe there are people with the potential to love us throughout our whole lives. Da loved me and I knew it, in the deepest place of myself I knew something unlike anything I had ever felt before. He had a certain magic, but by contrast he was my rock. I believed in him."

The next day, as Ellie and Suzan walk together, the tide high, forcing them into the softer sand, Ellie rubs the smooth pebble in her pocket from yesterday, the pebble that seemed to have helped her form the idea Maddy might come. She's encouraged by the progress her mother has made and doesn't realize by listening and understanding she has been effectual in her mother beginning to heal. Suzan has begun to eat; she sleeps well and rises looking more rested. Perhaps she stands long and in thought at the window facing the sea, but she catches herself and looks to find Ellie or finds a way to distract herself.

"Mom," Ellie says. "What will it be? Coffee or a nap?"

Suzan naps after having taken such deep breaths of the soothing ocean air. Sometimes, as now, she naps with Da's pillow folded against her stomach. She keeps the letter, his final gift to her, nearby. Da used to say that the memory of love will see you through. It's not so, she wants to tell him. The easy vivid recall of him in his coffin seeks residence and is paralyzing; the momentary disbelief is followed swiftly by the undoing realization that he is gone. And then again, he is there with her like a hologram.

Maddy arrives early Sunday afternoon, and they hear her shifting down the aging Honda half way up the hill. Suzan and Ellie are on the stone circular driveway to welcome her as she pulls in.

She is dressed in jeans and a large gray sweatshirt, 49ers' written in red across her chest. The sweatshirt drapes on her shoulders, big to accommodate large breasts that swell over her bra and obscure her figure. Unlike Ellie's well-kept car, hers is messy, chock full of papers, books, tossed clothing and whatnot. Suzan sees exercise weights in the back seat.

Maddy reaches across to present a round loaf of San Francisco sourdough bread in its white, red and blue sack. Ellie smells the yeasty flavor, feels the texture and hands it to her mother. "Remember how good it is?"

"Actually, I bought it in Crescent City just today. They must fly it in," Maddy says.

"We'll warm it up for dinner. Thank you. You must be Maddy." Suzan smiles broadly and puts out a hand.

Even though she's forty, Maddy has a youthful expression of joy, contagious joy, permanently etched in her freckled face. The color of her sun-toned freckles has turned her skin to light rust on her face and arms.

Suzan thinks that Maddy probably has an unending battle with her weight; it would be impossible not to with her short, compact build. Suzan has always had a bias against the overweight. She chastens herself for the thought, when obviously this woman is such a match for Ellie. Suzan is deeply relieved and welcoming.

To Suzan, Maddy turns, and says, "What a magnificent setting! Ellie has told me, but now I know why she dreams of being here. A beautiful buck loped away as I drove up through the pines, and now this spectacular view of the ocean."

She shields her eyes and looks west. At high tide, the ocean performs for her with dramatic swells and flourishing waves that leap against the rocks and, seemingly orchestrated, crash into the coves. They can hear its repetitive rush, a continuous roar, as it acts its part. Maddy takes a deep breath.

Maddy reaches for Ellie's hand, and they embrace. They release each other and embrace again. She turns to Suzan, "You've lost Da. I'm so sorry. From what Ellie has told me, he was a wonderful person."

Maddy has had her own practice as a skilled psychologist, but her aptitude is more a part of her nature than her training. She serves as chair of the board for a well-known rehabilitation center for alcohol and drug abusers downtown on Grant Street. Ellie's bank has responded to their proposal and has been instrumental in launching a new program designed for young men and women whose parents are paying for their rehabilitation.

"How do the adolescents get a stake in the game? The program needs to address that question," Ellie had said when reviewing the grant proposal. They met over the table in the bank and exchanged phone numbers. Within a day Maddy had called her at home.

By the hand, Suzan shows Maddy to the glass porch, and they stand side by side looking out to sea. Ellie stands back. She can see the silver in Maddy's red hair, tied attractively in a loose knot with an ivory stick through it. She aches to be held between those breasts. Who, but Maddy can give her physical comfort?

Suzan and Maddy's shoulders touch as Suzan points, "The sun will set about five thirty. Every day is different, but this evening, it should be especially beautiful."

Indeed, the colors will develop in the drifting strands, and the sun will illuminate the backs of the large dollops of cumulous clouds stacked on the horizon. It will be a cataclysm of color, flooding and blending. On any other given day, Suzan might have set up her paints in anticipation.

"I see now how it is that you paint such magnificent seascapes. The one Ellie has in her dining room draws me in, and I feel as if I'm there. Now, I am literally here, meeting you, Ellie's mom, the artist. I see, too, where Ellie gets her beauty. Do we have time for a walk before the sun sets? "

"First, let me show you Belle Haven…"

Maddy looks up to the cathedral ceiling and to the tower of windows. She touches the smooth ebony of the piano. Suzan tucks the bench in further, and they look into the expansive bedrooms, the natural light streaming in.

They walk down the beach and into the village, and Suzan shows Maddy the gallery where she sells her paintings. Suzan introduces Samantha, the owner, and she and Samantha talk easily together as Ellie and Maddy circle the room, hand in hand, remarking on each painting, standing back, getting closer. Ellie hears Samantha say how sorry she is.

As they walk back, Maddy lets her hair fly. It whips around her face and catches fire in the late afternoon light. Ellie's affection and passion is heightened by watching Maddy walk ahead of her, barefoot and free, an image she's not seen before.

A SEASON OF MISTS

They tie and begin roasting a plump hen. Maddy dominates with a sure hand. Ellie and Suzan are delegated to chop celery and onions. Suzan peels the potatoes and dices them, covering them with cold, salted water. As the memory of Da in the kitchen swims through her mind, she wipes her hands and touches the corner of his apron, the blue striped one he would have worn. He would have been sparked by Maddy's charm and energy. He might have contested Maddy on how to tie and roast the chicken. Suzan reaches in a pocket and finds his antique silver corkscrew. It shines as she turns it in her hand. She returns it to the pocket.

A glass of Sauvignon Blanc in hand, the promised sunset pulls them into the porch that frames the moving, changing picture. In the distance the cumulus clouds are stacked in flat-bottomed mounds, puffy and crowded, while the Sirius clouds stream ceremoniously across the sky, in various colors like a child's kaleidoscope held to the light. As they stand watching the transformation, Suzan looks at the empty cove being colored in as it reflects the drowning sun. She gasps, turning her back to the slowly changing scene, remembering Da dying before her eyes. The three embrace, and nothing is said. Ellie's hand goes to her shoulder. Suzan slips out from under and retreats to her room.

Maddy takes her camera outside and shoots several aspects of the sky. She points south and east capturing a sunset-bathed forested mountain cradling the sea in the distance. She situates Ellie for a pose with the sunset to her right.

The smells remind them, and Maddy bastes the roasting hen. The skin is crackling with golden, translucent bubbles appearing in the creases of the thighs. Composed, Suzan says, "What beautiful gravy we'll get."

"And it's chicken soup tomorrow," Maddy says.

Ellie washes, and Maddy dries. Suzan replaces the dishes in the cupboard. She moves Da's favorite cup to the back. The home is for Ellie and Maddy too, not just hers alone. And little Matthew will come. The future will be without Da.

"Maddy, you must be so tired. Why don't we call it a night? The bread from San Francisco was perfect with the roasted chicken. I loved the browned skin on the breast. I noticed you started it on high for a few minutes, then turned it lower. Is that the secret to keeping it moist and browned both?"

Much has changed for Suzan, and she feels dazed and exhausted. Leaving them in the library looking through the shelves, she realizes she is investing her heart in them as a couple. She likes Maddy. *There will be a child,* she says again to herself. She likely won't see much of Da's little Corrie and Dusty or the others now that Da is gone. She can't foretell, but she hopes the children insist on coming back to Belle Haven. Corrie has a budding talent as an artist, and Dusty loves the stars. She has seen he appreciates art. He's very sensitive like his father. His uncle Paul is his hero.

She handles Da's last letter, turning it over, looking for anything she may have missed. He liked to write afterthoughts in the margins. "*Je t'adore,*" she finds in the margin of the last page. On another he has written, "forever in love with you." He said it so often. He never tired. Her heart is softened toward him as always.

Finding fossils

The following evening, seated, looking toward the dark sea, their chairs not facing each other, Suzan begins to talk. "The time I met Da for the first time, Ellie, I had you and little Matt with me. You were a year, and he was four. I was leaving Africa because of a kidney infection, even though our term wasn't up. The three of us were going from Abidjan to Paris then to Switzerland to see a specialist recommended to me. The plane was hot and crowded. I was bogged down with all the baggage: blankets, bottles, diapers, and all. The stewardess led us down the aisle. A man, Da, it was, stood up, commenting: 'The whole damn family?'"

Ellie says, "That doesn't sound like Da."

"He spoke in French, but not with a French accent, nor was it American. Perhaps he thought I wouldn't understand him, but, yes, it was a grouchy thing to say. We were getting off to a bad start, especially for a crowded, overnight flight.

"I ignored him, and didn't greet him. I settled in the middle while Matt sat in the window seat. We were all so tired. I had left you and Matt with a friend's daughter, while your dad and I went out to dinner with the other missionaries just before our departure. Because I wanted to give you a bottle and get you to sleep early on, I asked the girl to not give you the bottle I had ready. You must have gotten fussy, because the bottle was empty when I went to get it from the diaper bag.

"You threw up that whole bottle of curdled milk she had given you. Fortunately, I had a baby quilt around you, and I could make a little skirt of it to catch it all. Da reached over and we wrestled the quilt out from under you. He took the quilt away, and the stewardess disposed of it. I undressed you down to your little bare back and began to put your pajamas on you. You wouldn't remember the ones we used then; they covered your feet and buttoned down the back. I loved those pajamas. You were a sweet baby. You liked to cuddle.

"When he returned, I thanked him. He brought wet paper towels, and we made the best of the situation. He took off his sweater and put it over Matt, and he looked so much more comfortable. The plane had gotten cool. Finally, you went to sleep in my lap. Motioning to me, he asked if I would like to put you under the seat in his foot space. Using the pillows and blankets from the plane, he made a little bed for you. He transferred you down and patted your back when you stirred. You slept the whole night through.

"After the meal was served and people were settling in for the long flight, and the lights were low, I touched his sleeve, his left sleeve with my right hand, to say thank you. He leaned over and said, 'May I?' and kissed me. Here was someone who knew my anxiety and put himself out to help me with you children. I was so touched. I returned the kiss, and it felt like the first kiss in my life. When our eyes met, I saw a man with a great passion for life, and something more. His eyes expressed an admiration for me I had never seen in a man's eyes. His kiss was slow and gentle.

"We talked and talked, and I told him my heart about the marriage, how trapped I felt having been committed to those fundamental beliefs all my life, but now doubting my purpose in life. I even told him I didn't think I was a Christian any longer. There I was, married to a minister.

"He told me his history, how, as a teen, he had to avoid being caught by the Nazis in the Netherlands where he grew up. When they invaded in 1940, he was seventeen, like ripe fruit, ready to be plucked. He would have been sent to the work camps. Instead, he was able to attend the university.

"Marrying, getting a scholarship, coming to America, he completed his doctorate in Agronomy and another in Statistics. I asked him what agronomy meant, and he laughed and told me he was a farmer.

"He told me that he and Cora, his wife, had agreed to never talk about their Judaism or the invasion of the Germans into the Netherlands with their children, or anyone for that matter. He had feared for his life every day. At one point, he had hidden in the country on an abandoned farm that had been the home of Jews, relatives of Cora's, who were already deported. Cora and he conceived a lie of sorts, a lie of omission, never exposing their children to the truth of the cruelties they had experienced. The children didn't know their father was beaten three separate times. Neither did Cora and Daan talk of those times between them. That awful chapter was closed. Cora never regained trust in humankind. Her world stayed very small.

"I was very vulnerable, Ellie. I was twenty-five. There was something about him, the attention he gave me, the value he put on my thoughts and feelings, something magnetic. I've never doubted that I fell in love with him during those hours."

Ellie shifts in the chair, and the soft leather creaks as she turns toward Suzan. Suzan turns, and Ellie holds eye contact with Suzan, saying, "Everyone is vulnerable when it comes to love, but you were more so. What were you, nineteen, when you married Dad? Matt came when you were twenty?"

"I have never confided in any one about this, sweetheart, but not until Da and I had physical relations many years later, did I understand what I had missed. Determined to succeed in the marriage for you and little Matt, I dug my own grave emotionally those twenty years. I had never explored my sexuality before marrying. I knew I was missing out but didn't know to what degree. If not for you children, I wouldn't have had the will to stay as long as I did…

"Ellie, I know it isn't fair to criticize, but your dad didn't want anything to do with you as children. My illness in Africa seemed like a nuisance to him. I often felt we were in his way. It was an old familiar feeling. He had never changed a diaper, hadn't ever rocked you. He didn't read to you or Matt. I was already alone, so early on. My own parents had thoroughly enjoyed each other. I just thought it would be that way for me too.

"Our goods were held up by a dock strike, as was our Land Rover. We only had what we had in our suitcases. Nonetheless we went to the bush and rented a small house to begin a new work there, to build a church. Soon after, the Director of Missions asked your dad to go to Ghana to help at the press. He left us there in the desert, and it was a turning point in the marriage. I began to understand we weren't his first priority. We had no transportation or running water. I hired someone to find food for us each day.

"You've heard this Ellie, but I repeat it because I have never told you the experience in the desert was a turning point for me as a person. I was determined to make it. I had clothes made in the market for you children and me. I could have gone and lived in the mission guest house, and no one would have thought anything about it. Instead, I was proving something to myself. I stuck it out. I've never regretted it. Something good came of it: A new sense of self and my own strengths.

"He only returned every few weeks for a day or two. There was always the danger of the border crossing between Upper Volta and Ghana being closed. If a coup were to occur, we would have been separated for a long time. A lot was going on with the Biafran War in nearby Nigeria at that time. As it was, a bribe had to be paid to get across into Ghana and out of Ghana. Otherwise a person could sit in the heat for hours. If you were bringing a sack of flour or sugar, they often took it. After that year, your dad was asked to move to Ghana, never mind what was invested in my endeavor in the bush. We had no choice but to go with him.

"After those experiences, I determined that I would finish college as soon as I had the opportunity. I did once I was back in the States, even though your dad opposed it. I borrowed from my parents and went anyway. It took me a long time to patch all my transcripts from various places together. I ran that little weekly in Scotts Valley for a while after I finished. Then I went looking for something more secure. Your dad was unable to support you after the divorce.

"I couldn't have ever become a civil servant, writing for the Air Force without that degree. Within a year and some months, when we divorced, I had the security of the job and health insurance for all of us, something we hadn't ever had. I know, it's unheard of in these times to be without insurance."

"But Mom, Matt and I, we became more and more aware as we grew older. We understood, Matt and me. He wasn't at our games. He didn't hear our speeches. He didn't go to the beach with us. I don't think I ever heard him tell a joke. Maybe it all had to do with how he grew up, but we knew as teenagers he wasn't a regular dad. I remember he missed my graduation from the eighth grade. Seems silly doesn't it? I knew he was very smart, even brilliant. I admired how he could do the exegesis he did for the courses he taught."

"Da wrote me the first letter, just hours after we parted that early morning. He always found me after that, even though we moved several times. When the letter came, it was like a mirror to my own feelings. I returned his letter, owning my feelings, and sharing more or less how I was faring. I don't have those letters. We corresponded from 1970.

"We began to meet soon after I divorced twelve years later, and after a time we found Belle Haven. It's been both our retreat and our home. He leased it for us for several years, and we bought it after we married. Except for the remainder of yours and Matt's college funds, there wasn't much saved, but I helped pay. He knew it was important to me to be part of buying it."

"Mom, are there any letters left at all? Ellie stands and looks toward the escarpment. She is framed by the stand of trees on the half a mountain lit by the nearly full moon, the sheer, striated face of rock delineating time, layer after layer, century upon century.

At the mossy base, Suzan and Da had found gray, split marine fossils with whole shells intact, and they marveled then about the effects of time on the planet, the hundreds and thousands of years to move mountains and oceans and forests, and then to think how long it took for humans to evolve. While time affects humans irrevocably, they cannot affect time. Looking at a cliff like that, one senses his detachment from infinity.

How was it that their illegitimate prayers had been answered? Perhaps they were not as sinful as they believed in the context of such a timeless universe. Does the passage of time eclipse our sins? Do they fossilize and stay hidden? With so little evidence one can only postulate their history.

As Suzan continues, Maddy remains quiet, with a stillness of spirit, a reverence for the mother-daughter exchange. Professionally, she is trained to remain unaffected while a client expresses feelings, but she feels now a different feeling than that of a professional. Her own mother died of breast cancer, detected too late when Maddy was sixteen. She is drawn in a daughterly way toward Suzan, especially because of her openness with Ellie. She feels as if some of her own needs will be met through knowing Suzan. Maybe she'll feel less like an orphan.

"The letters left are from 1982 through '84, something like that; they're some of the letters I kept after I left your dad. Da and I were just beginning to see each other when time allowed, and we agonized trying to find our way forward. It's a bit of the history of our struggle. Finally, we came to terms and stopped agonizing over whether or not what we were doing was right or wrong. We found this retreat, Belle Haven."

"Will you read them with us?" Ellie asks.

"Ellie, the letters would be too hard. You'll hear our joys and pain, and how deeply we cared. I'm sure we explored our feelings way too much in them, but I want you to know him Ellie, so you know whom I've lost.

"No, you may read them together, but I don't want to read them again just now. You can use the library, and I'll begin sorting Da's things. The advice is to do it soon after the death."

Suzan brings the letters, removing them from their myrtle box, laying them carefully in Ellie's lap. His letters have been written on most any kind of paper, old bills and receipts, even a napkin. Some are on his personal stationery or from the office. By the contrast in their penmanship and uniformity, it's easy to tell them apart. Suzan wrote on blue paper with a blue fountain pen. Comparing her ability to express herself to him, she always believed her letters lacked chroma while his were saturated in full color.

The smell of the myrtle is akin to a freshly-sliced cucumber, clean and pungent. All have been correlated in chronological order one on top of the other, the first to the last.

"Perhaps, these will open windows for you."

Down by the sea

They sit closely together on the floor in front of the fire, legs stretched, the collection of letters between them. Before they begin, Maddy touches Ellie's face and says very simply, "I love you."

"And I love you. Maddy, everything is changing between my mom and me. We've talked, especially about my teen years. Even though she's suffering, she wants me to be closer than I ever expected. She wants me to know her. Some of her stoicism is going away, and she's not isolating herself."

Maddy chooses to read Suzan's letters while Ellie reads those written by Da. Suzan hears the murmur of their voices going back and forth. Painfully, she begins to sort the sweaters, the shirts, feeling and seeing the worn sleeves and collars of his favorites. As fastidious as he was, he couldn't let them go. His suits, forty-four regulars with a thirty-six inch waist vary from grays to blues. The obligatory black, shoulders shielded in plastic, had been of little use. So distant from his colleagues, Da and she rarely attended funerals. He tied his own bow tie when in his tuxedo, and multi-colored ribbons drape forlornly on a silk hanger. She sorts by piles to go to Goodwill, or to the Mission in downtown Portland.

She catches when Ellie and Maddy are silent and hears the murmur of their indistinguishably quiet exchanges. She hears affection in their expressions to each other. She wonders if they'll be put off by the affluence of words, the stretching of hers and Da's soul as they try to articulate. She feels a kind of nakedness allowing Ellie and a stranger to read her thoughts from nearly twenty years ago. She will hear the teakettle whistle or ice being dispensed into their glasses when they take a break. She will fall asleep before they finish in the morning hours.

Maddy begins to read aloud:

Santa Cruz, California
January 11, 1982

> Da, when my thoughts turned to you during the night, I didn't really imagine that you might be thinking of me. Even though the phone beside me was not yet connected, with no possibility that you could even know where I was or how many tears wet my pillow, comfort came just by the thought that had you known, you would have called; you would have understood.
>
> When I finally decided, and began the search for a place, then actually moved, nothing could stop my eyes from filling with those most unusual tears. I cried at the slightest provocation, and all day Saturday, as I said before, they flowed, warm, relieving me of any bitterness I felt. I felt as if I were being bathed in grace.
>
> I wept with sadness too, for David, the beautiful, good man he is, and for what I have always known we could have had, had we known how to get there. I have always worshipped him; he's extremely intelligent (a scholar in Greek and Hebrew, a star among the faculty) and informed. I have envied those who receive his best. He is loved by his students and the faculty members, but is a stranger to his children and me.
>
> There is so much to say and write. I have been nearly paralyzed, unable to hope at all. Now some clarity comes, and a deep peace, some confidence in my ability to make good decisions, patience with myself for the ones I make that aren't so good. That painful yearning to get back in touch with one's self and produce from the core of one's being is the very essence of what has prompted me to move out of our home. I must find my way and find meaning. I didn't feel impulsive, but I felt a slow coming into my own, an eagerness, yes, but

pacing myself now to write and experience my thoughts such as they are.

There are times in our lives when an inexplicable reawakening happens, and it began for me the weekend I saw you. After being with you I could not put away the desire to expand back into being me. The person that I am and the 'me' I am becoming won't differ in quality or character, I hope, but only be strengthened and enhanced. How could I have ever given up the helm of my own ship?

This spiritual rebirthing is indescribable, beginning with you, in its earliest stage when we met for the first time in 1970. I've benefitted from your love and your aspirations for me. Some of Pascal's idea hit home right now, his defense of the Christian theology. I just want to become who I'm supposed to be.

The actual resolution to move came by contrasting the sense of fulfillment I had that day with you so recently and the immediate sense of deprivation I experienced upon return. The culmination of all my deliberations came, when I found this apartment. A great calm came over me when I began to work out the details. Somehow, you're a part of it all.

Support came from my assistant. We moved in several hours. I am so grateful to her. David stayed long at his office, and it was late evening when he returned to find me gone. I couldn't have handled him knowing beforehand. He would have physically blocked my way.

Spiritually, I don't feel thrown out of the 'garden'. I realize the portent of God's question to Adam in the garden: "Where are you?" Is it possible for you to believe as I do now, that Adam was not called to answer for his sin, but was being called back to the habitual communion they had shared?

My hiding from Him, and you, has been because of my misery and my sense of failure and guilt, the feeling that I was powerless to woo David to share a more emotional and spiritual bond with me. I think this restoration to fellowship without David has been God's goal all along. I held to his coattails for so long. Am I egotistical to assume God wants my communion? I am alone in that sense of fellowship, not conjoined. I believe the choice for communion is always mine, whether I stand or fall, whether I fail or succeed. King David of the Psalms certainly floundered, but continued his relationship with God, pouring out his feelings in songs and prayers. I'm sure I will waver in my thoughts about this.

I had a dream. I was standing atop a mountain with a stranger, an engineer whose specialty was building roads. He pointed to several roads that lay in the forested valley, twisting and going nowhere, it seemed. He asked me if I realized why the straight road he then pointed out was straight. He proceeded to show me how it turned abruptly right, leading to my destination. "Follow the signposts. Go on the straight road. This way, much of the strain is relieved from the traveler. You've been so confused, you're exhausted," he said.

I woke in the morning with a sense of wanting to make it easier for myself. The big picture is hard to get when surrounded by the trees and underbrush of a forest. Such a ridiculous over-used metaphor. I do believe I make things harder for myself because I doubt myself so often.

I saw *Gandhi,* the film. Perhaps I was ready and received all the more from it because I have studied Christ's life. I've never listened quite so keenly. I came home with a renewed decision to be true to myself. (May I say here, I love you, and that is being true to me. I feel allowed to hold you, physically hold you.)

A SEASON OF MISTS

The apartment has the most serene setting, a meticulously kept garden to which the whole living room is exposed. It's beautifully lit at night. I can see birch, cedar, climbing ivy, rhododendrons, bonsai, fern, Monterey pine, and jade. My desk looks out on to it and I feel content. The ocean, its sounds, and the magnificent, ever-changing sight of it are half a block away. I love the exquisite quality of this little neighborhood. Those tears purged me, and an infinite tenderness bathed me, perpetual and sure like the waves breaking on the shoreline. It seems as if I compare everything to the ocean!

I've wanted to say so much more. I am open to your love now. It's awesome to touch the spirit of another. Come, be with me for the span of time reality will allow.

Thank you for your letter. Thank you for understanding my sense of renewal, and with it a permission to love you, something for which I know you had prayed.

I love you, Da

Suze

January 12, 1982
Sunday evening

My dearest Da,

I am finally in the apartment with the children, having moved only yesterday. I took very little, only three beds and two dressers and various other things and had completed the move by one or two in the afternoon. The purchase by and by of a few pieces of furniture will be all I need. I have been looking for just such a place for some time. I finally found this unbelievably perfect place, in a meticulously kept, old part of Santa Cruz, just near the yacht harbor and a half block from the shore. A doctor and his wife own the place and occupy the apartment above me. I have a lot of security and a very restful atmosphere, with a Japanese-like garden in back. I can hardly wait for you to come. I can receive you *here* in my own environment after these many years.

Yesterday was the most emotional day of my life. It was if the fountains of the deep had broken up – my face streamed with tears nearly the whole day. I believe I love David and am moved with compassion for him, and all the doors are open for our reconciliation, but I wish I could describe the marvelous peace I have, having left him. If only you were here, I could experience you in a whole new way. Here are two letters in one, saying the same thing essentially: that a whole new chapter is beginning.

Your Suze

Washington D.C.
Friday, January 18, 1982

My dearest, sweet Suze,

I started my annual leave two days ago, that's to say the day before yesterday. I spent all day paneling the laundry room and yesterday, I was running all over town with my son Paul, who was here for one day, taking him from one appointment to the next – mostly with Senators and the National Dairy Association.

We own dairies together. He is good in the dairy business and has done better than I ever hoped. He's become an expert and knows more than I. I took Paul to the airport early this morning; spent already one hour in my office to clear up a few things I left half-finished on Wednesday, and now, before doing hundreds of chores in and around the house, I have taken refuge in the World Bank's library, where in a quiet corner between the stacks, sheltered from prying looks and incommunicado to the many colleagues and investment officers who all want my advice, I can finally devote myself, without pressure and without feeling guilty for doing it on the Bank's time, to writing to you . (Now, wasn't that a terribly long sentence?)

What better way than starting my real vacation to write to you, my beloved?

I have been under great pressure again to perform at the office. Even though I have been back for more than three weeks, work tends to pile up. All the data I collected must be sorted out and ready for presentation.

In Peru, the cattle are being bred to adapt to high altitudes. They're artificially inseminated by bulls in Switzerland. It's quite a program, using prize bulls, shipping the refrigerated sperm into the heights of Peru. Although much time will be required for the entire herd of the project to be affected, the lung capacity of the new cows and new calves is remarkably increased. The cows are actually producing more milk, and even a little cheese operation has developed. They use mules to transport and distribute the milk. (I would like you to see the site of the project, the beautiful views of this green, irrigated valley from high up. One sees waterfalls spout out of the side of the mountain.) Do these particulars interest you at all?

I expect this project to look as good on paper as it did when I was there. I'm over my head in work, yet my colleagues who find me in my office assume that I am readily available to chat for hours with them and if I don't close my door, (which is glass) I won't get anything done all day.

In the meantime, I keep looking out for a free moment to write you, but instead, have to be content with composing a few nice phrases now and then, which I usually have forgotten entirely by the time I sit down to write you.

So, you'll have to do with whatever words tumble out of my mind.

As always, I have been thinking a lot about you. As Father Brown (of Chesterton's stories), I am trying to put myself into your skin and follow you through your daily routine at work and at home, from the moment of getting up after another restless night, thinking about all the things needing to be done, wondering whether or not you made the right choice, feeling the greater burden of caring for yourself and your children, and the next moment rejoicing about the newly gained freedom, to make place again, in turn, for the agony of loneliness and craving for love. Then at work, there's some relief because the pressure is on, hundreds of things need to be attended to, things have to be straightened out because of misunderstandings among your co-workers.

How ever did you agree to start up a newspaper for this Indian fellow who calls himself a developer? You'll have to keep him out of the editorial page! He has to be put in his place, and you wonder how you can do it in the most tactful manner without upsetting him and therewith your own apple cart. At least you have health insurance.

I can only imagine the excitement you must feel and joy you are anticipating, or will being single suddenly crush you with its weight of loneliness? Who or what will fill your life then? Will it be a complete fulfillment?

Oh, my dear Suze, I can imagine the agony you must be going through, the burden of choices, of decisions, of reactions. Life must be hell at times and I hope to God that there are at least moments or stretches of moments during which peace descends into your heart and you can relax and face the world with renewed vigor. You know that you still have a rough road before you, but you also know you can manage, and, by God, you'll make it.

Forever, Da

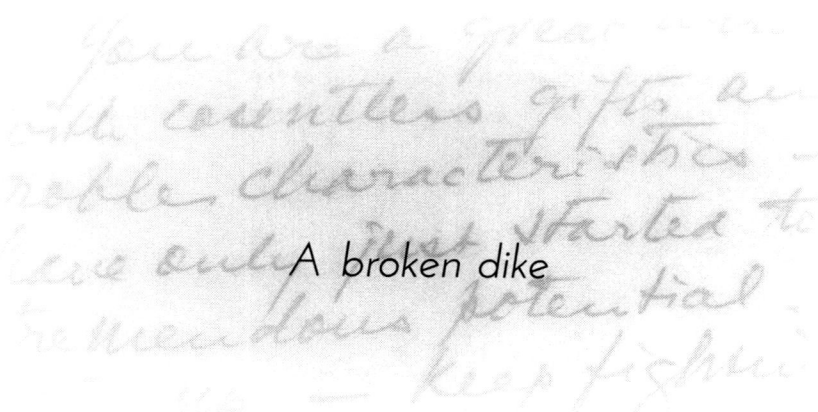

A broken dike

February 2, 1982
Santa Cruz, California

Dearest Da,

Someone to whom I've spoken from the recesses of my heart through the years. Again last night, I lay awake talking to you, feeling you understand. Everything is changed for me, Da. I'm finding gates to the dimensions of my soul.

How much I would cherish days with you just being and sharing, then, finally, returning to families, circles of friends, expectations of others. I feel I can come to you freely now, without hesitation. As opposed as you seem, I have gone forward with a divorce. It seems the only way I can survive. My perceptions have been correct all along, though I've rejected them many times, trying to get past them. I knew it by contrast, when I met you, Da, and now these years later there's no reason to hold back.

Da, from a distance, since moving day in January, I feel scarred from these years of being married to David. I feel as if something huge has been lifted off me. I'm resolute to be true to my own intuitions and gut feelings from here on out. But, so much time has slipped away. It's mid-life for me, bringing me to say an emphatic *yes* to your suggestion of a week, a weekend, a day, some block of time, allowing us to plumb even further the rapport we know, and have known, through corresponding. The longings have lived on in spite of separation, so much change and some of the trauma of living in Africa another three years after we met, even as you managed a tea plantation in Kenya. We were the breadth of a continent apart, yet I had the expectancy that you might visit or call or write. That expectancy never left me since the night we met.

I look directly into the mirror, and I think I see a woman now. I am at least appreciating me as a person. I am more protective of my love for life, not to allow all the regrets overwhelm me. I feel more trust in my own decisions, especially as I succeed at work and in other relationships.

Because of the separation, I can no longer work as a development officer at the college, so I've agreed as I said to start up *The Valley Times*. The school paid very little but it helped. I shouldn't have accepted the offer, but then I didn't know I would have the courage to actually leave him and my whole world.

Yes, I have taken on the job of managing a new, local newspaper, here in Scotts Valley for a developer. There are eighty acres of beautiful property that lie in a valley. I will sketch it out for you so you can see how beautifully pristine the valley is. He very much wants to sway public opinion in his direction. I only agreed to the job if he agreed to stay out of the editorial page. Of course, those in his camp are taking out ads in the paper while others don't even want it thrown in their driveway. Growth or no growth? Acting in his interest, I've spoken at the city council about the zoning to allow the growth, probably not very persuasively. Anyway, it's a job for now, and he's paying me well. I have found a managing editor. I hired him because he's so very handsome, and you should be jealous.

Thank you for your perseverance and acting to preserve the memory of us, our kindred spirits, our communication when I felt too frightened to be responsive. I felt scared to be loved the way you seem to love me. Shall you always love me, Da? I'll always love you, because even though I have held another, you were always part of me, since the beginning, since that night.

You remind me of a winter wren, a small songster I remember from the Pacific Northwest. From such a little bird (only the males sing) comes the mightiest song that rings through the woods. And one hears the competing arpeggios. Your mating call can't be outdone by any other. Your songs are liquid, complicated and long, and beautiful beyond measure. Did you know the wrens have two sets of vocal chords? You must have at least three.

Your beautiful year-round wooing is complemented by your gentleness. When the night got cooler, that first night together on the plane, you covered Matthew with your black wool sweater. I remember your kindness to me, and your shoulder, when I slept briefly.

Matthew may be a poet at heart. At sixteen, he loves words. He doesn't excel in math, even though he works hard at it. (He was four that night on the plane.) But then not everyone can be an astronaut. Ellie is a little trouper, a bit competitive for such a pint-size. She'll probably have a growing spurt, now that she's thirteen. Da, they were babies just a day ago.

I remember you remarked on Matt's beautiful blond hair. It's still blond. Looking at mine, you asked if I have Norwegian heritage. I told you that the children do – their father's father was an immigrant from Norway and David is very proud of his heritage. I'm just a mutt. Now, you wouldn't recognize them, but you have found me once again and still hold a torch. Maybe you'll come to know them.

A SEASON OF MISTS

Since our last long dinner (that luscious baked red snapper) near me here in Santa Cruz at the harbor, before the separation, I often imagined you alongside me. Now I have a new permission, and I take you with me for long beach walks. I scuff up the sand with bare toes as if beside you, laugh as you ruffle my blowing hair, lie naked of soul and heart with you, stroke your chin and nose, letting the awareness of time slip away until the aura that surrounds us when together (and permeates our letters) brings us into its flow again, wanting to recapture and retain those awesome feelings of meeting you and connecting in the almost magical way we did. I want more than your hand across the table.

How fragile, and preciously guarded, is that overwhelming oneness. I know it is ours again, even if I, with my anxieties, seemed to have yanked it from its roots last year before it flowered. Perhaps seeing you last year even though I gave you a flat out no, prompted me to separate from David. Come again my love, or let me come.

I know that you know that when I went back for my degree it was against his will. During our waking hours, I was corrected; my spontaneity killed; my ideas rejected; my advice ignored; my opinions disregarded. No other person has ever hurt me more or as often or as needlessly as the "man" of our house. I steeled myself and didn't react, thinking it would all change. Now I can see how it has been one long fruitless struggle for me to please him.

At least I have my bachelor's in spite of him. Now I see how I just stood there, too dumb to do anything except try and please him "according to the scriptures." You know, a "woman's place" in this sub-culture in which I've been reared and married into. As I succeed, I am even more threatening, and his attitude is accentuated. (I got a good bump-up in salary). I feel foolish to have waited for permission to go back to school. I feel foolish, period. I might as well be my mother, subservient, but oh so necessarily devious at times.

I have always wanted time to talk and laugh, and play together with him. I've watched other couples with envy. We've never had a vacation.

I heard some words from my sister, words I needed. She tells me my family in general has seen his incapacity for relationships. They have seen his absences, his inability to play any role but that of a disciplinarian for the children (and me). He began spanking them when they turned two. (I think it was a minister named Dobson who wrote a book, giving that advice.) My parents will be supportive, even if reluctantly. Divorce is against their beliefs.

David's self-righteousness (or is it a lack of confidence in himself masked as such?) leaves me with no other choice. I grieve over the lack of true companionship. I want friendship and equality. I was nineteen when we married. I thought it was God's will to marry a minister who wanted to go to Africa. Da, I didn't know about loving someone or being in love. What path now? Because of our denomination, he can't be divorced and teach at the college. We both have our challenges. He will resign.

Enough said. You can see the importance to me that you wanting to know me became, because I am not known, and intimacy isn't really the intimacy I imagine it could be. How terribly important your letters, your expressions of love have become. You love me, all un-put together, having blundered my way into your heart, coming to you, spilling my tray of doubts into your lap (or was it the baby who spilled on you?) To this day, you love me even as you mop me up.

I want to know you, have time to explore the tide pools here in Santa Cruz, whole worlds unto themselves, to let the changing of the tides pull at the sand around our ankle-deep feet, time to explore the complexities of who you are, time to share about pain and dying. I want time with you because I love you. You should watch Matt from the shore as he surfs in. Although Ellie doesn't surf, she loves the sun. By the time summer arrives, she'll already be tan. With her blonde hair she'll look the part of a California girl.

Suze

P.S. Here is something I wrote last year before my decision to leave David, about the coming of spring and some of the pain I felt entering a new season, not having made my decision to leave. Do you like my attempts at poetry?

> *To muted atrophy*
> *Edging into the middle years,*
> *To a spring-widowed shadow sighing*
> *A skeleton's song,*
> *No lids to fasten the eyes,*
> *Who, seeing, sings the modified whimper of wasted*
> *Yet sensing flesh,*
> *Flinching at promise.*
> *Crouching beneath the eaves,*
> *Grieving again the departure*
> *Of winter's shrouding sameness,*
> *To her, spring comes*
> *Like the unpracticed knock*
> *Of an unknown child*
> *Who bears no good.*

Spring came to me that way last year. Rather than respond to it, I crouched in fear. Now, I've made a decision, Da. I felt out of touch with nature, not in harmony with the singing of the birds, not eager to turn the soil or pot a pot. I felt the loss of having been insulated (hidden) during the winter, with all its shadows to shelter in, it seemed. In the startling brightness of spring were only those remaining shadows under the eaves. They evoked in me a sense of abandonment. But after such a long period of indecision, I've decided to save myself.

P.P.S. Have you had to dig out from that terrible storm, so late in the year? I imagine the snow is heavy and wet.

"There seems to be a gap here," Ellie says, reaching for her glass. She stretches out full length, leaning on one elbow in front of the dwindling fire, and then rises to put on another log. She smothers the fire completely.

"Damn," she stuffs in more newspaper, but it flames out not catching the new log on fire.

With the poker, Maddy rolls the log back and arranges kindling and paper beneath it. The flames conflagrate and lick the bark and begin to burn steadily. "You know in my practice, say, when someone is going through rehab, they write some of the most beautiful stuff. I can almost hear your mom speaking that beautiful verse. There are lots of people who react to the seasons or holidays. People often die on a special occasion, like a birthday or at Christmas. They also can become more depressed or unsettled. I wonder if she's doing any writing now. I hope so. It would be good therapy for her if she were to write a journal. Listen to me talk."

Maddy is both professionally and personally evaluating Suzan, and the lines are blending. She reminds herself to not be a coach, just Ellie's partner.

"In these letters, her hopes are tied to Da."

"There's a certain magic to their bond, a real gift. They had hope. In his mind, she was his constant companion, an ideal maybe. But neither is being exploited."

Sometimes, it's better to have a lingering, nearly smothered hope than no hope at all," Maddy says. "Although, according to a Psalm in the Old Testament, 'Hope deferred kills the soul.' Thank God they survived their own earnestness."

"This next letter only has page two." Ellie turns it over.

"Maybe the magic is the distance between them, or their age difference, or something unearthly to dream about and revel in."

Faces flushed from the warmth of the fire they move into the recliners on either side of the hearth.

A SEASON OF MISTS

London
January 1982

My Darling Suze,

The time will come when I should disappear out of your life, something I know already, but find difficult to face. However, as long as I don't hear from you to the contrary, I'll keep writing you in the hope my letters give you a little joy and peace of mind.

Just before leaving my office this morning, I put in my official travel request for a month-long trip to South America, starting mid-February. The projects there vary from new vineyards to coffee plantations. They are effectively self-sustaining, always my goal. This, my dear Suze, is why I continue this work, nor could I stand being at a desk all the time. I plan to do some business in New Mexico and California, before flying to Bogota and, if all goes as planned, will be in San Francisco some days in February.

Will I see you? Shall we plan to consummate this terribly beautiful tie?

I'll be thinking of you, my love, as always. I love you, you know that. What you may not know, is how much I love you…

As ever,

Your Da

London
February 21, 1982

My dearest, sweetest, loveliest Suze,

If you only knew how often and urgently I have wanted to write you, ever since we said adieu at S.F. airport and how I desperately tried to find a way to call you and couldn't. Whenever I took paper and pen, ready to start a long, long letter to you, I found I just could not. I still cannot honestly let myself feel, because I am afraid I may get carried away and write, blurt out, my feelings of love for you in such a way that this temporary shelter we tried to build ever so carefully would be undone with the stroke of a pen, so to say. I can't explain it, but I can't leave her, Suze.

Later...

Suze, you have been in my thoughts, constantly, persistently, a constant bittersweet, but oh, so precious, reminder of our glorious twenty-four hours together, our first. Why have we waited over these twelve-plus years? I have talked with you during the many hours of trans-Pacific and across South Asia flights, during the hours upon hours of being jostled in a van or a jeep through miles and miles of plantations, while walking the streets of Bangkok and Kuala Lumpur – hot and sweaty – throughout meetings (very, very boring and tedious sessions with even more boring colleagues). Whatever I did, I was thinking of you, and reliving the rare excitement and sensuous pleasure of just beholding you, of seeing you as you are, giving yourself to me, every second and minute of the twenty-four hours we spent together. The joy of holding you in my embrace, of enjoying your physical and mental presence – of literally having you to myself.

Oh God, Suze, I love you, I love you, I love you! If only I were younger. If I could do it all over again – life, that is – I would not hesitate to marry you.

When we parted that Sunday afternoon, I felt like I did when I was a child, dreaming that someone gave me a beautiful present, and then just when I was grasping for it, eagerly with both arms, hands and heart, the dream faded away and I woke up empty handed. I had the same sensation, when I saw you drive away on that bleak, colorless stretch of the Pacific Highway and only the thought of hoping that it was all to the good, that this is what you had to do. That is, return and resolve to re-make the marriage as I encouraged you to do. Nothing kept me from crying, for I knew there might not be a next time, that I had probably lost you there and then and forever. And, strangely enough, I prayed that that was the case for I, Da, what can I offer you instead? Nothing permanent, nothing solid – only very temporary solace and satisfaction (and even the latter is perhaps doubtful). Still, I can understand why you will try again with him.

Close to the surface

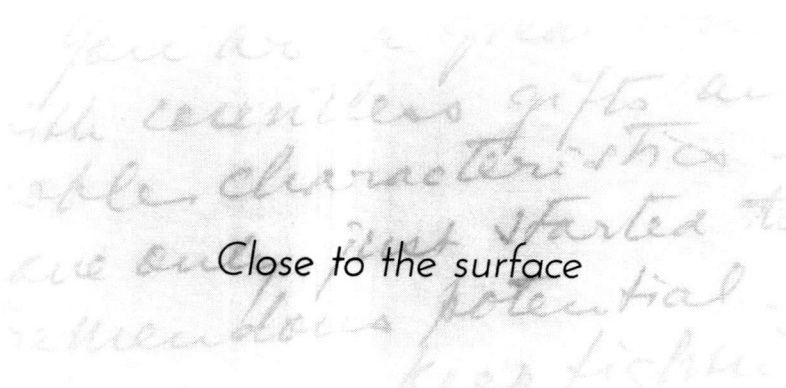

6 March 1982
Hilton Head

Suze!

Wish you were here. Thought of you a lot, and did a lot of just meditating, while making long, long beach walks by myself, gradually trying to reconcile myself to the inevitable, i.e. seeing you again in this new way. I've not had a lover, have you? How does one manage? A dike is broken inside my soul.

Slip out of my life if you must, the hurt is there, but the pain is easing somewhat because I know it will be best for you. I still hope to see you in S.F, just see you and talk with you. I am not asking for great promises or can I make any. Will you see me again? I am looking for a place for us.

Love, Da

P.S. I'm in Harbor Town (Hilton Head Island, South Carolina). Flowers are always in bloom around the harbor and town houses of this Sea Pines Resort. Harbor Town is one of Hilton Head's most unusual attractions.

A SEASON OF MISTS

Undated
Santa Cruz

Dearest Da,

I have opened the letter I wrote you just after seeing you. It is so disconnected and poorly written. I will start over and try to convey what it wants to say. A week has passed since I saw you. Your love is like a cradle for my swaddled, helpless feelings.

On the weekend, Ellie and I took our first sailing lesson. Out there in the swells, I wondered that I didn't feel afraid, just exhilarated. I played several hard sets of tennis and had a lovely brunch at the famous Shadow Brook Inn. On Monday, I drove to see the counsellor in S.F. I think it was beneficial and probably the last time. How can one know what these doctors think, but he seems to nod understanding of my decisions. I talked with him about you, your intention to meet my needs in some way.

A famous roller coaster here in Santa Cruz is just across the lagoon on the boardwalk. At night I can hear the screams of the riders, always when they hit the peak of the ride and pitch down, experiencing the pleasure/fear. In my fear, I'm feeling an excitement for life that wasn't there before. I'm on the roller coaster and heading down and maybe I'll crash. But I'm exhilarated.

I miss you, and yes, I will marry you, or did you ask? It felt as if you did. The counsellor helped me see that I can't keep waiting for David, and that the discoveries I've made are good. I'm up against someone who is very guarded and insulated. I can't tear down all his defenses, or, as the counsellor said, I would leave him in pieces.

All my love,

Suze

August 3, 1982

My Da,

I have read your letter so many times it looks a bit frayed. I'm sitting in what looks like a chateau in the now defunct Santa's Village investment property owned by my employer. The sunlight streams in my upper story windows, opened to the freshness of the morning air. I feel alive and refreshed this morning, and that perhaps accounts for how beautiful the setting seems. The Redwoods' shadows pattern those tempting paths, a kind of invitation into fantasies of childhood, when one's imagination was aided by all the potential in life and growing up to be... ? Growing up to love...?

The other day, as I raced the tide in and chased it out, feeling that child alive in me, I imagined flopping breathless beside you in the sand, closing my eyes and giving myself to your presence, the absolute complement to those feelings, going from playfulness to arousal. Just now, here, the delicate designs of dancing sunlight through the breeze-touched oak, remind me of how time seems to stop, the mind stops babbling to itself, and only the presence of the other matters, just as the coral tones of the room in San Francisco complemented or enhanced the sweetness then, not at all like an ocean setting might have: the wild beauty of the waves mounting and crashing. We'll have that too. But the soft touching of discovery, the fear and wonder, being absorbed without consciousness of need, a basking, the conclusion is unneeded, unsought, taking you in because you have finally released yourself to experience me and I, you. Out of commitment to ourselves, we have held back over these years. Yes, I would love a place of our own but, how can we manage that?

(When I hear of plane crashes like the Pan Am Boeing that went down in Louisiana, I can't help but worry about you.)

A SEASON OF MISTS

August 4, 1982

Da,

It is another morning, in my loft-like office, still, quiet, and the dew waltzing like white fire in the trees.

Yesterday, I was watching the birds while lying in the sand at Natural Bridges alternately beating their wings and gliding in the wind… rising as they resisted the hurtling wind and sailing forward when they released themselves.

Stewart Emory has written a book entitled "Actualizations", which impressed me. In it, he talks of never being able to be on course but always staying mindful of the destination, like a sailboat tacking. And so we make constant adjustments, nearly always off course. But that does not preclude that we won't be able to get to our goal – namely, being ourselves, actualizing our potential.

Similarly, as I watched the smaller birds, the chubby marbled murrelet and the rough-winged swallows I saw how they make use of the wind. Often, they fly so close to the surface of the water, their wings beating so fast that they're unaffected. I think our problems and challenges can be seen as like that constant buffeting by the winds of the sea, which resisting doesn't help. Nor does it help to try escaping them, nor does the rejection of our efforts to be free of contrary forces. So often, I've compounded my inability to cope by despising my humanness, while acceptance with a sense of accountability for my humanness actually augments my strength and moves me forward.

My letter to you, unfinished and tossed, upbraided you for settling for an environment that disallows you being you, that is, your marriage. After receiving your letter, I see that you know that, and I'm glad at least that portion was never mailed. The book I made reference to helped some things gel. I'm not where I want to be, but I feel confident the errors will get corrected along the way. Tacking, constantly tacking, as we did on the sailboat, me at the tiller.

Fear can settle in as quickly as the fog rolls darkly over the hills of the Bay. Remember how that happened in Half Moon Bay, how it rolled in as we watched, that black, moving bank, looking almost like smoke, while smelling so sweet? Changing the air? Then, it was a cloud of contentment that enveloped us. Now, I'm keenly aware of needing you, feeling hopeful but so scared. Da, I feel scared.

I will paint Half Moon Bay as we saw it, the rows and rows of pumpkins beginning to mature, the vines sprawling in the lanes, the stretch of sea just beyond. Remember the place we found with the African art near me here? I bought the two Bambara Chiwaras primarily used in Mali to seek blessing on their agricultural endeavors. They're sitting on the mantel and remind me of you, my dear farmer; I'm praying that your agricultural endeavors succeed.

How sensitive we are to when we cross ourselves, such as your experience while away and alone. You're not alone in that. Let go of the shame. I know you're human. Sometimes I think we must experience those times when we're unfaithful to our inner values in order to move toward "actualizing."

What a beautiful and hopeful compliment that you sense an inner unity while with me. What more could I want to be other than one who provides an environment that nurtures who you truly are, to experience you translate the images of sound to art as you choreographed our love-making to Rachmaninoff's third, to see life in your face and a comfortableness with your body and your sexuality?

Rollo May, the author of a book about the will, points out that facing our demons releases us to be natural. I guess I'll have to face them one by one and not all at the same time.

The ache for you to be you is part of me, because I am investing myself in you, the natural you. The unpolished, imperfect you is the one I love. You are vulnerable, receptive, and responsive when with me, maybe sometimes even like the pouting disappointed boy you referred to. The quality and longevity of our relationship depends on how many of the pretentions fall away, yours and mine. You aren't old. When I am seventy, (you'll be ninety) I hope to still be me, a twinkle in my eye, a sense of daring, not succumbing to a no-risk life devised out of survival techniques. That seems so long from now.

You've been schooled to continually reject your feelings. "C's" reactions to you are equal to rejection. My God, Da, come as you are, if you come to me. I can't forget your face turned to me, telling me of an earlier time in your life in the Netherlands, when you overcame so many obstacles while being afraid for your life. Time hasn't changed our affections. Twenty years between us is not a chasm we can't cross. No, it is rather to my benefit, the fact of you finding me time and again, at last with your heart in your hand, mellowed, even more gentle. I love the lines in your face.

Time gives gifts, which more than compensate for our losses. There's the deepening of love and the increasing mystery of it. I'm in awe of your genius, your knowledge and appreciation for the finest in life, your worldliness, the strength of your passions translated into words. Let me cry when it is you who touches me, or as I yearn to unite with you again as we have.

So fragile our spirits – Adam knew Eve and Da knew Suze and with that knowing, that act, comes an atmosphere of total acceptance. So know me, in every sense of the word, because I love you. Know me as in that poem I wrote you, "Love me to love me":

> Love me when a winter's night
> Has persuaded you to claim my body
> For warmth against the cold.
> Love me in frolic when a summer's night
> Has freed us of all our covering.
> Love me in a meadow, or on an orchard's floor
> In springtime when the earth is fertile
> And life has charmed and coaxed you into its cycle.
> Love me. Turn in sorrow; turn in silence
> When there's drought and there are no buds of promise.
> Let me wait with you for the flood
> of newness, sure to come.
> Love me when day is dawning,
> And your passion for me has mingled
> with your passion for the day
> Don't mind to take your leave,
> The same day dawns for me.
> Love me on a rainy afternoon
> And read me verse as I sit beside your chair.
> Love me when music has stirred you
> And some beauty convinced you
> To respond in some way to something living.
> Love me for pleasure; love me for need;
> Love me to love me.
> Love me with tenderness; love me with disregard.
> Make me laugh; make me groan.
> Make me know you, your ways, your heart.
> Make me your own.

Da, never go out of my life.

When we were together, and I was touching you, you said, "You did it." I was taken aback because my intention was not to have intercourse again but to give you pleasure, however I could. You must understand I am not measuring how you do. Nor do I want to wear you out! Seriously, I want you to simply experience, on this new ground, that I love you and welcome you. Welcome me into your heart with its turmoil and conflict or into its serenity, whatever you're experiencing. You honor me to love me... to listen. I'm a comrade of your wandering soul.

Love always, Suze

Maddy turns the page to see if there is more on the back. "Do you remember your mom seeming depressed? Writing to Da seemed to give her an outlet. What do you see, now that you look back?"

Ellie looks away. "All I can say is that she must not have acted the way she felt. To me, she seemed so strong. We always had her great cooking and a lot of attention. She was always more tender to Matthew than to me. We didn't share many feelings. She expected me to do well in everything, but she let it slide when Matt couldn't do algebra for instance. 'So you won't be an engineer,' she said. I'm going on, Maddy. I've never really talked about my childhood to anyone. I've told you about loving Sonja, but I could never have told her. But, no, to answer your question. We were all so busy with our own schedules. She didn't seem depressed. She was my mother."

Maddy strokes Ellie's cheek and pushes back her hair.

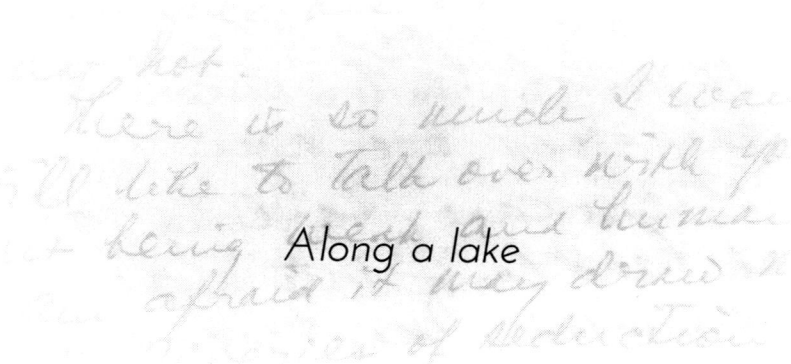

Along a lake

Swiss Air
Geneva — New York
August 12, 1982

My dearest Love,

I had to make a quick trip to Khartoum again for about a week, and you were there with me at the confluence of the two Niles, the White Nile and the Blue Nile becoming one and flowing toward Egypt, a beautiful metaphor for our coming together. Together we are a new river, changing course forever.

How I would love to take you to the botanical gardens here. I am on my way back to the U.S. again. Swiss Air is taking good care of me, as usual.

My love, my dearest Suze, I have thought of you, daily, nightly, hourly, whenever I am inclined to escape this harsh world of reality, of pressure and discomfort. I think of you and think of all the things we might do.

In the Sudan, in Khartoum, electric power was out most of the time (there was some sabotage at the power plant), and we sat through long, sweltering meetings, and, at night, I couldn't sleep because of the semi air-conditioned state of my room (working on standby diesel power of the hotel).

A SEASON OF MISTS

And so, I turned my mind to you whenever I could– I have held you in my arms.

Truly, you are my constant inspiration and my constant delight. Again, I am probably doing a dangerous thing, writing you as a lover. Unlike before, while not really knowing where we stand at the moment. How will it go for us?

I certainly hope that I will find the promised letter in my box upon my return. How disappointing, frustrating, and dispiriting it can be to trot back and forth to the post office, day in and day out, without finding anything in that little square opening.

Suzan, my love, my inspiration, I spent the last eighteen hours or so in Geneva, mostly walking – first *la rive droite du Lac Léman* and the Rhône, next *la rive gauche*, finally the old town – searching for you. I moved back twelve-odd years in my mind: I just left you at Orly in Paris, you were destined for Geneva, if I'm not mistaken. Finally, now then, I have come to Geneva. The weather was gorgeous – warm and sunny, (it must have been typically Swiss-foggy and drizzly when you were there), your image was firmly imprinted in my mind. I kept on walking and walking.

You know I am not kidding. Time and again, whether I walk in Washington, or Bangkok, or Khartoum, or Paris, or Geneva, or wherever – time and again my heart skips a beat because I think I just saw you passing by. I stop in my tracks, turn around as fast as I can and follow that familiar figure only to be disappointed. Often, it's the build of the girl I passed. More often than not, it's the curly hairdo or the side of that soft face with the cute little nose barely visible.

Old Geneva played funny tricks on me again. Give me any old city in Europe, and I am going through a time machine. I am almost beginning to believe in reincarnation. I have been here before, I keep telling myself, not this century but 100–200 years ago. I feel home again, and very, very nostalgic for what it was once back then.

Oh, my dearest love, everything I saw and experienced these last eighteen hours in Geneva was with you. We walked along the lake and I commented, reveling in the calm of the next green easy flowing park near the science museum, backtracking through Rue de Lausanne, along the Rhône finally, marveling at the intense peace of the priory (rather, the remaining foundations of it), at the very end and yet still well within the city. This morning, working our way through the clouds on the narrow pier, leading to *jeux d'eau* looking up at its enormous height, spraying waves like a giant flag, a brief respite in the Rosaria in the park at the *Rive* lying in the grass, in the shade of a huge and ancient tree, planted by one of my ancestors, surely a nobleman. Reminding you, while tickling your face with a blade of grass, how we once made love in the woods. I'll never forget the whiteness of your slip, which you kept on, giving you a virginal quality, which scared the heck out of me, then.

Finally, my dear Suze, we stood on the little square adjacent to St. Peter's church in the heart of the city, this morning listening to the tolling of the bell in the tower of another church, only a few hundred yards away. I was holding you close to me, whispering all sort of promises in your ear, telling you, "Wait until we meet some day or rather some late evening– a moonlit night on the Campidoglio in Rome (which Michelangelo never saw finished) gazing over its many hills and valleys and being captured by its fascination, as the old emperors must have been when returning from their battlefields, in victory, with the assurance that God was on their side.

A SEASON OF MISTS

Last night, in the so-called famous Richmond Hotel I did not sleep much in my three by six meter "maid's" room with barely a breath of air to cool it. It was hot and uncomfortable with those lousy, soft, wavy beds in Europe. My thoughts kept turning around you, as ever. I find myself developing a strong split personality or, at least, a split life. My thinking and spiritual life revolves around you, you only and my active, physical life around my job and home.

Can I go on this way? Should I go on? Is it fair to you? To her?

In all fairness, I would not necessarily marry you. I'd rather run away with you, travel with you, go beachcombing with you, find peace and quiet with you, just be together – be whole, be content, feel young and indestructible, ready to live an eternity. I'd buy a picnic basket.

I have made arrangements to meet the realtor on the Oregon coast, where we last met. What a wonderful place it was. You could even drive there on your own. I think it's a hopeful lead. I know how you loved the place and that part of the world. You can paint there, Suze. There's that room that would be perfect for a studio.

I love you, and I find I need you more and more. My life is not complete, not whole without you – unbearable.

C'est la vie. At this point there's nothing I can do about it and neither can you. I just cannot leave her. She needs me too much, and she has over thirty years invested, so to speak. We were teens when we married and had Paul.

I wish it were different but there you are. I love you, worship you, adore you. Anything you may wish or think of, let me know. Perhaps a place of our own will be a solace to you.

For the time being, the only solution I can think of is the same temporary arrangement we have had in the past. A one or two day visit, now and then. It's better than nothing at all, at least for me. But how about you? Will you continue to go for it? I'll try to lease Belle Haven, that place we love. There is where I first saw you in moonlight, surrounded by the sound of the sea. I feel as if I'd like to plant a flag on that 'half a mountain' as you call it.

Please say yes – because I love you and miss you.

Forever yours, Da

September 3, 1982

My dearest Suze,

I know you are as busy as I am, especially since it is a new job you are doing. I fervently hope it goes well, and have no doubt it will in your very capable hands. How is it being a civil servant?

I miss you terribly. I have read your last letter so often, I know it by heart. As you say in your beautiful way, I will love you to love you! You are still constantly in my thoughts. Whatever I do, I think of you, ask you what you think of it, compare notes, and observe your reactions.

When driving back from work each evening, I am in a state of euphoria, driving my new Cadillac Eldorado, and listening to the most divine music on the radio or from my very carefully selected tape collection, while the wind through the open sunroof blows my hair and hot brow. That's when I hold lengthy discussions with you, or imagine you resting on my shoulder or lap (as you did in California).

Suze, if you only knew how much I love you!

A SEASON OF MISTS

I gather no amount of writing will make up for our separations but at least it fills the gap a little. All we can do is wait, wait, wait and then we'll be together again. Maybe for only one day, who knows? But at least that day will be bliss again. Yes, each time will be better than the last time, for gradually, we will begin to know each other's habits, likes and dislikes. I do know you love me too, and I am overjoyed in that knowledge. I believe you have an understanding of my feelings for you, as well as my appreciation of your feelings. As you know, I am a very sensitive person, and nothing escapes me. Even though we tried hard to be ourselves our first time, there were some little skips now and then. Understandably, considering it was the very first night together, and we had to cram all our emotions, happiness, agony, ecstasy as well as our sorrow and grief into such a short time span. Now we are flowing together, as naturally as nature itself.

I do know you, as Adam knew Eve and make no mistake about it, I love what I see, hear, and feel. I love you, all of you, body and soul. I worship you my love, as I have never worshipped a woman before.

You are the gist of my life, the tonic my spirit and body need, my inspiration, my hope, my Love!

Since I talked to you, there have been some changes in my travel plans again. Both "C" and I will be leaving on September 14 for Holland, where we will have some vacation until October 3. "C" will then return to the States, and I will continue to Turkey alone, from where I shall return mid-October. So, I shall have a chance to write you. How about writing me, if only a few lines, before I leave on the fourteenth or else upon my return? I long to hear from you. After Turkey, I will meet you, hopefully, in mid-November.

All my love, Da

Adrift

September 14, 1982

My Da,

What is it one does when one has sinned against herself? There's no one who could understand my aloneness in this. I feel so unsupported, and I've left the only world I've ever known since childhood: the denomination, colleagues, family, friends. I feel holed up, not wanting the responsibility for myself and the children, or adrift like flotsam; my self-esteem and confidence are gone, and life seems so meaningless. I'm nearly thirty-eight. Why am I here?

I want answers, but can't conceive of where to go to find them. If they lie within me, everything is too murky to dredge them up, and I'm not sure it's worth the effort. Oh, for the day when my mind will let go of what's troubling my spirit. Most of all, I want to be guilt free about seeing you while you're still with Cora.

Are there answers in the church – in believing? Shall I redress my faith? Ask, no beg, for forgiveness? Or is it a boundless sea we live in and our faith only a makeshift barge, unseaworthy in the end? Is it in this crude fashion we hold off coming face to face with reality: that is, we are in this all by ourselves? Do we already know this reality and are too afraid to face it?

Somehow, I just cannot go back to my fundamental upbringing without having to change my basic self. And yet, it is undeniably a part of me. I need you. I have to let time lessen the pain of my transgression.

Love, Suze

P.S. I wish you were my Boaz, that I, Ruth, could lie down at your feet and be covered. But I'm no longer sure God has His hand in our love for each other.

Swiss Air
October 16, 1982

My dearest, loveliest Muse, my Suze, my source of inspiration,

Again, in spite of all good intentions I couldn't get to writing you earlier. I hope you received my KLM air letter mailed from Istanbul on the fourth of September.

Again, I can finally begin to relax, knowing that I will be in this airplane seat for the next six to eight hours without any major distractions in the offing.

Again, I am bone-tired, having worked literally around the clock since last Sunday: In the daytime I was visiting farms, livestock auctions and those awful slaughterhouses, plus smelly sausage plants and rendering plants which stink so bad that the smell stays with you all day long and night, unless you scrub yourself raw.

And again, at night I had to work up the data into financial and cash-flow tables which kept me up until three, four or even five in the morning. At seven, I had to be back up for the next field visit.

Yet, I won't complain. I still love this job. The World Bank has been good to me. Each day is another adventure. Sure, there are not many that come without minor problems, or big ones, or even real hardships but I keep meeting new people, seeing new vistas, letting my brain absorb new ideas… and no matter how old I am, I still find a lot to learn. Life is just too short. I try not to think of the day when I will have to call it quits.

When I leave the World Bank and retire, I'll probably go on consulting and have a go at it again, at least part of the time. If I have to stop entirely, I'll go crazy and probably follow the advice of my old geology professor: "Can you imagine," he said, "to be a geologist all your life and to die of old age? It would be far better and far more glorious to just fall off a mountain peak at the end of a strenuous expedition." The poor guy, he did, after all, die in bed, after having had cancer for more than a year.

Suze, my sweet love, it occurs to me that I am writing you my memoirs; so to say to you, my truest love, having arrived at my door. What's more you are the only recipient of these. Your responses are a lifeline to me.

Formerly, I used to write my impressions of trips and missions, either in a diary/notebook or in letters. I have an old broken-down atlas I keep, where I have marked all the places I have visited and worked. On one such page, in almost illegible pencil I have marked where and when we met.

I don't have the time to write everything twice, so here it goes, to you alone! It is a two-way street really. I feel the need to express myself on paper as you know and on the receiving side you are such a wonderfully willing recipient to take it all in.

After all, you are my Muse!

Turkey was quite an experience. My colleagues and I crossed it from west to east all the way to Erzurum, not far away from Mount Ararat while we saw and crisscrossed the Aegean region, out of Izmar, which, by the way, used to be Smyrna named after Queen Ismyrna or something like that. Standing on the balcony of my hotel room, the very first day and looking over that glorious bay, bathed in sunlight, with ferryboat, tugboats and tankers crisscrossing it, and the hills around it, with their Greek and Roman treasures scattered all over them, interspaced with the ever-present minarets, signifying the location of a mosque – that glorious morning, to be followed by many mornings like it. I will send you some shots as soon as they are developed. Then and there, I dedicated my heart and work and thinking to you, my Goddess, my Suze.

As usual, I have done a lot of thinking on this trip, coming to the final conclusion that life is too short to expect to savor it all. That became all the more apparent when I stood in awe of the maps at the various museums we visited, both in Izmir and Istanbul, showing the spread of the Roman Empire until about 400AD, and the expanse of the Ottoman Empire many years later. To think of it, how those individuals got along in those early times under the greatest of hardships, with primitive forms of transportation and without any decent map to speak of. (Here I go 500 miles per hour with a modern map, cursing that it does not have the details I am looking for!)

Of course, we must remember that the poor foot soldiers probably didn't get that far or live that long. They were dispensable – in the country they were cannon fodder or more appropriately "arrow-fodder". If they had to fight, or if they had to fight a foreign war, they were herded onto a rowboat or something larger than that. If it sank, oh well, there were others who would make it. No helicopters were going out to pick up survivors, that's for sure. I'm rattling on about how the common man might have fared.

I'm not planning to give you a lecture in history (actually one of my weakest subjects, but one which fascinates me greatly)...

Anyway, I have a feeling I am going about it in the wrong way in my thirst to see the world. As I said before, I have a large atlas, way out of date, its pages becoming very fragile. It still names Stanleyville as the capital of the Congo, for instance. I've penciled in all the dates and places I've been. Only one entry is personal... I've penciled in ever so very lightly in the margin, *February, 1970 met Suze*. No one reads this old beat-up book besides me. I have been to almost 100 countries now, worked in about sixty to seventy and I am still searching. Searching for what? Truth, wisdom, beauty, peace, rest? Frankly, I don't know. You alone, provide respite.

I do know that I could find great delight to just sit with you somewhere on a wall in the country, on a rock, on the ledge of an escarpment, overlooking a valley, being on a shoreline or sipping tea or coffee on a boulevard in Paris.

One doesn't feel that far away in Paris, yet your body is at rest, your eyes, ears, and nostrils take it all in – seeing, tasting, smelling, hearing, becoming one with it – and yet I keep it all at arms-length, so I may be able to describe it all someday or should I?

Why not become one with it, love you entirely and openly, and inject some of my own feelings into this life? So what if I become emotionally involved? What if I left her? Oh, Suze, I can't think of it. I simply cannot.

I have taken a break. Oh, Suze, I would like so much to be with you, to write something worthwhile, beautiful, good, not so that my name may be counted amongst the great but just so others may have a chance to participate in the emotions I feel – those fantastical, almost spiritual feelings you get when you stand on top of a hill, the world far below you: huge, gray curtains of rainclouds hanging in the distance, a titanic battle between the almighty sun and armies upon armies of cumulus clouds, trying to obscure its ray and shaft, keeping you spellbound. Oh, forget it!

Just when I am moved to the ultimate ecstasy and am beginning to believe that I am capable of great things, it hits me like lightning from those same nimbus clouds that here I stand alone, naked before my God and His creation. And I am only one, just one of the billions of people in this world, a good percentage of whom may have the same impressions. Why should I be the one to have the freedom to love you freely or write something which feels to me to be unique to us?

Who would read it, other than those who are very near to me (out of curiosity or compassion)? Besides, I know my shortcomings, my lack of grammar, my incapability of coming out with properly structured sentences. A few days from being fifty-eight, I guess I am a little too old to learn.

The long and short of it is that I am beginning to feel myself leading a very selfish life. Yes, yes, I am sharing it with others but they're only too few. My children were participating in it when they were still home. Now that they have their own families, they don't seem to care, really.

She, "C", shares in it and somewhat affectionately, I am sure and yet, most of the time we are miles apart. Strangely enough, we both have an inborn shyness, which we somehow never managed to shrug off in these many years together. We had a little vacation in Holland and England… but it is you who is my muse and inspiration. No matter what we did, you were always by my side. I am torn.

So, there we are – a pretty unique relationship. I suppose I am a dyed-in-the-wool bigamist unless it is actually a stronger power forcing me. I am not planning to give it up. I want you and I love you. You have become a part of me, inseparable, at least in my mind. I cannot make any promises… you know that… All I can say is that I deeply love you and that I share a closeness with you I never felt before with *anyone*, including my wife.

I now hope we will have a chance to get together soon, very soon. Are you still coming to Washington? There's so much to talk about. What is this about transgressions? You're the purest soul I know.

All my love, my dearest, one and only Suze.

Forever yours,

Da

P.S. I want to take you to the new EPCOT Center in Orlando.

October 17, 1982

My dearest Suze,

I am sorry I have no birthday card to send you but herewith goes a part of me: my heart, my love, my thinking… it's all yours. I can tell your spirits are better. That was a snag along the way, whatever it was that was troubling you, and now you're back in the stream floating more peacefully.

Happy 38th Birthday my love and many happy returns!

I send it with the hope that we will at least share some of our life together.

A SEASON OF MISTS

I love you, adore you, worship you as my goddess and for this occasion would very much like to hug you and kiss you. Happy Birthday, Love! Forgive my lack of stationery!

Your Da

October 22, 1982

My darling Da,

I lay awake again last night talking with you, pulling you to me, imagining my breathing in keeping with your own, perhaps because I was moved by the letter and the call – so rarely do I hear your voice. Yesterday, my birthday, I was able to read the letter as if you were speaking it. The stirrings are sweet, sweeter now for the assurance of your love. The end of my day is *my* time, though I, too, think of you throughout the day.

Finally now, the letters are you, so wonderfully you, the sensitive, tender, gentle you, one who embraces his world, its people, its grandeur. You and the physical world come together, and I love you anew, more deeply now, in awe of the man I now know. Your letters have a new quality, an openness.

How beautiful the moment when I unlock the box and see that familiar handwriting. One day, I had to delay reading your letter and kept feeling the expectancy well up. When things slowed down, the letter was there, a gift. I treasure you more at thirty-eight than at twenty-eight or at twenty-five when we met, when I thought I would explode if I couldn't have you near me. I know now the lifelong experience we'll have. Now there is no either/or. I do have a sense of gratification and closure even though you are so rarely in my arms. Perhaps one's values change, but each letter is as great a gift as any man could give a woman.

Thank you for sending the key to Belle Haven. I think we should keep the name, *n'est-ce pas?* I want to paint that tossing ocean before long. Can you come mid-November? I never want to be there without you.

My love, you *should* write; you're gifted with a passion for life. You are how one should be in this world, feeling it all, seeing and experiencing in a broad and grand way. And, if you can't begin to write, then let us say that your letters to me are the beginning of whatever you want to communicate, to wrestle with: conflicts, responses, fill in the historical context of your trips, their purpose, and geographical significance… whatever.

Then, if you wish, when my file has grown fat, we can arrange to have them typed; you can edit and create from them the format you want. I will be your memory keeper. I've always said to myself I could write with inspiration if I were writing it for you, Da, because you have at times pulled the best from me. Any dialogue you may want with me is fine. I'm quite unflappable, and anything you ever think, you can say to me.

I love you, your human feelings, like how you tramp the face of the earth with such diligence, searching, wanting to experience it all. Da, my Da, you're both brave *and* afraid. Courageous children, we are, to explore our own minds and entertain our own simplistic questions. Those hovering questions are like living angels who flutter about us. They are pure, simple, inevitably unanswered except by inducing more questions.

If I could unleash my passions just now, I would smother you into unconsciousness just to see the wash of peace on your face. (Hopefully, you would recover.) And yet, it is that milky blue, searching look in your eyes that compels me to keep pressing for you to disclose yourself to me.

A SEASON OF MISTS

The mystery of your own honesty leads you into hunkering down with despair but sometimes elating with labile, all-over-the-place expressions of joy and exhilaration. In some ways you're like a Thoreau – you could contribute so much to so many because of the way you see and describe. Was it Faust who in German says: jubilating to the sky and depressed to death? That's you.

You, my love, owe me and others someone with whom to identify through your writing, not in a dominant tone of either agony or joy but the true-to-life way you live. I identify with every motive, pure or impure. Your greatest gesture is that willingness to spiritually consummate – clumsily at first, but gracefully, at last – and we do consummate spiritually as spirits may do, without encumbrance as we let go of our inhibitions and let go of what we think we should be doing. All to say, yes, you should write. You may write to me of other times of your journey, even when succumbing to despair, self-love or self-hate.

Sunday evening

At last, some time. There is soft rain, the house is quiet. A German chocolate cake rests on the counter for a belated celebration a little later. It's just dusk. I'm also thinking of Monday morning and all it involves. Already you've probably begun to think of retiring and how your Monday mornings will be slow and easy thereafter. For now I have this time with you.

It feels good to have a good bout in the kitchen, folding in egg whites, melting chocolate. I wish we shared daily living together. I've given thought to your desire, and mine, for me to be with you more often. Then, of course, there's the reality of our Belle Haven, hidden away. (I loved your Steak Diane.) It keeps my hope alive.

I can't bear that we should give up sharing being together; give up allowing this intimacy to be integrated into the whole of our worlds, a fully rounded-out experience, among others, but together. I would walk so proudly by your side. I'm stumbling along, just to say, I wish we were a couple like other couples.

We are willing to compromise this dream, but my ultimate dream is to be with you as you describe, letting the intimate moments creep up on us while overlooking a valley or peering into a shop window in some remote, faraway place, but in an everyday way too, Da. I can't run away, Da, not even with you. However, I'd like to be in Rome with you, just for a day.

Will I ever know the world the way you do? I want to say take me along and "teach me" and also to say "listen". My own learning and growing is of value as well, even as a relatively untraveled local here in California. My journey is bumpily spiritual. Sharing it with me I'm sure is very jostling, like the washboard roads in rural Africa.

As for the job, I can't observe others without empathizing, and sometimes, I've had to retreat to save myself pain or to keep from making a poor decision. Managing people as I do now exhausts me, but it is fulfilling too.

Yesterday, an older woman called to tell me I am like a fountain from which everyone drinks. The obligation of meaning that to someone makes me uneasy, and I do want to run. Detachment is impossible. And so the learning goes on as people bring me into their lives and disclose feelings and thoughts. Now, if I can discern how to respond. I have secrets I will never share, a conscience that won't be appeased. On to other things…

A SEASON OF MISTS

I miss the newspaper. We were a small team, but we were a team. Putting the paper "to bed" on Thursday nights was almost a party, laying it out, watching the columns fill up and then getting it over the hill to San Jose to be printed overnight and delivered the next morning. Sometimes the typesetter was cranky. I purchased a second hand back-up, slower but reliable. I made a practice of ordering pizza on the house since we were always running late Thursdays. We delivered the *Scotts Valley Times* on Friday mornings to about 7,500 homes.

(Later)

I find refuge in the fact, in the security that I am loved in such a beautiful and meaningful way by you. Some kind of filling up takes place as I read or reread a letter or think of the way you hold me in your inner sanctum and the way you gain speedy access into mine. I love that we can retreat to Belle Haven, even though it's like pretending. Remember Dr. Zhivago? The isolation, the beauty?

Now, if some day we may interpret this by our living either by writing as we do or by loving well in the many other aspects of life. I, too, want to write. I'd like to tell our story.

I remember a very long time ago I had a vivid dream; the memory and comfort of it is still fresh. I woke with the sense of your presence all around me. In the dream, you were in the kitchen making breakfast, and I was waking up in a soft, downy bed. Wide doors were open to the very green, wooded countryside. There stood a grand piano in the most beautiful setting, sword ferns all around it brushing against the ebony, moving slightly in the breeze; it was just waiting for you among the flowers and shrubs. Maybe it was Forsythia I saw, because I remember the yellow.

The prevailing sense was of comfort and pure joy; an unqualified satisfaction associated with your presence. Remember playing for me that late night in the lounge of the hotel? You're very gifted. I suppose you sing as well! I'm going to paint the scene in my dream of the ebony piano against the beautiful overgrown garden. But, not you. I could never capture who you are with my paints.

I feel more fully integrated into the world, away from the constraints of my old beliefs. But an ache I wrestle with is to live up to my own potential to write, I suppose. Someday. What is it I want to write?

My darling Da, I know you understand what I am describing. From his father, John Milton inherited the luxury of opportunity to be formally educated. I wonder, in all his suffering, if he ever considered the greater suffering he might have had if he had been deprived of learning Greek, Latin, Italian, and on and on, studying all the works set before him, his writing an expression of his intellectual inebriation. I wish for tutors to make me wise and prolific.

Time has gone by too quickly. I've not nearly opened the tide gate we referred to so long ago in a letter. I wish I could snatch those capricious, fleeting words out of my unconscious to identify and communicate feelings. Metaphors play out, never standing on all four legs, as they say.

Let me now, as I close, hold you in the crook of my arm, smoothing your face pressed against my breast, as

> *I lay my hand on the soft shell of my womb*
> *No closer to its mystery.*
> *Twice swollen, it cushioned*
> *And nourished in darkness,*
> *Children... unknown, unnamed...*
> *And threw itself into convulsions*

A SEASON OF MISTS

To deliver them to the day,
Stretching me to receive them.
I move my hand,
Cup it under yours
As you lift my breast.
The sun is rising upon us,
The engorged bosom of a new day...
Cupped in the hand of a beloved.
Strands, fingers of clouds,
Pillow and plump the readied nipple
In the cavity of a cumulus palm.

Run your hand along my thigh slowly, letting the longing well up in me until your face is a blur, until I'm restless to cover you with kisses, until we know no other time or place, only each other and we feel the absence of the alienation (we all feel) and even by all these letters try to abolish. Come love me again with my innermost part open to you even as you penetrate my body.

I love you, Da

Suze

Sea change

28, November 1982
Sunday afternoon
Hemet, California

Da,

I have just come from the hospital. I stayed with Aunt Sara through the night until just a few moments ago. I feel as if I have been in a dream, holding you one night and holding Aunt Sara, so frail now, the next. Crying some tears in an empty cafeteria, adjusting to the shock of seeing her so weak.

Darling, I must tell you, I looked into the mirror quite accidentally, and I saw a woman of integrity, softened by compassion, and I met my own eyes in a new way, with deeper understanding, acceptance, and a more all-encompassing patience.

Aunt Sara needed me through the night, the old bond was rekindled and made stronger by the reality of death she faces. Congestive heart failure is a terrible way to die.

The fear and pleading in her eyes brought tears to mine. That deeper wisdom of hers returned as she dabbed awkwardly at my eyes with the corner of her sheet.

A SEASON OF MISTS

In a way, the depth of our communication is more profound because she can't speak. I seemed to be able to guess many of the words she tried to form, and that brought pleasure to both of us.

She didn't want me to stop reading from the Gideon Bible (New Testament and Psalms) I found in the drawer. There was a sense of assurance as the old feelings returned – my love for The Word, that familiar book. So I read Psalms 61, 41–42, 91, 139 and then from John Chapter 10, 14–15, 17. I also read the last few verses of Matthew 11 during the course of the night.

If I am any judge, she has two to three days. I will be glad for her.

Thank you for meeting me at the Hyatt. It was as if you were still there for a short time after you left. Like before, the book you gave me seems to have been chosen for me, exactly where I am. I left the room soon after you. Uncle Jim arrived early to take me to the hospital, so about the time you were boarding, I was adjusting to what lay ahead. I stayed a day and a night. I read until he came to the Hyatt to get me, and I read more between 3:00 and 6:00 a.m. at the hospital as she slept.

I remember a moment in the a.m. as I held your head against me, consciously in awe of you, wanting beyond words to impart something of my love, even as you slept.

Beside you, I slept so soundly, the fears dismissed. I was nearly sick with fear. Fear, now stated, has been that you would trifle with my affections. I've not been entirely willing to feel as I did those years ago.

Friday night, I felt a trust that I'd not experienced, living with a man as I did who was not my friend, who wanted to hold me back, even my education. I want you to know I wasn't afraid that being with you would equate to a (California) mudslide or an earthquake, because I'm facing the fact of this affair head-on.

Although I have not finished Pascal's writings, some things come together now. Being with you is a gift to me, a huge risk that has been amply rewarded. I feel so tender toward you — oh, the welling up in me, remembering your touch, your gentleness. More than lovemaking, I want to hold you and absorb who you are. The Mahler (it's so long) last weekend seemed to prepare me for the night with you and for this new level of love. I'm not squirming in doubt.

I have had a nap now, gone back to the hospital and fed Aunt Sara her pureed dinner and am ready to sleep. My eyes burn, but I wanted to write you. It's already late, and we leave for Ontario at 7 a.m. I'm still working for Mr. Sari on the side. I've appointments in Scotts Valley regarding the property when I return to California. He's trying for a third mortgage, so all the lenders have to agree. My moonlighting job has become multi-layered.

I hope you have recouped from such a long flight. I'm in love with you and am comfortable with the increasing strength of it, glad now to yield to it, as one confronts a truth that has already been a part of the subconscious.

I have a fantasy of riding with you in a taxi in a big city, perhaps a feeling that can be associated with that long flight to Paris… the beautiful tension of passion unreleased and building. We must always create a prelude for our times together — find ourselves at the top of a skyscraper, at the end of a pier or on a merry-go-round stretching for the brass ring. This is how I people you and me in my dreams. While you are my joy, I can know you better in the context of the world we share. Why does the back of a taxi seem romantic?

A SEASON OF MISTS

You speak of aging, less now than when we last met at Belle Haven. I feel pain when you do because you associate it with the pain of losing your attractiveness to me. Not so, and I shall prove it.

Loving you is not a lark. We make a memory to pull out of the hat later, and then we go along our separate ways. For years, we have returned to our relationship, (always your doing) and I'll pay the internal price, now. My softest flesh, my most vulnerable self is bared again. We are not common lovers, but maybe we aren't the exception. I don't know of anyone who has spoken of the rightness/wrongness of the pleasures I feel, nor of the pain when separated and deprived. Your letters keep the balance tipped your way.

Who are you, that you should claim such sacred ground in my heart? You can count, now, upon my being as foolish as before in order to taste the wine of your love one more time, for I am wise enough to be...

Your fool,

Suze

Ellie picks up the next letter, but Maddy stops her with her hand. "I remember when my aunt was dying. We had been really close. One of my first memories was when she came years ago and teased me about missing my two front teeth. She seemed tuned into me. She told me about my menstrual cycle well before it happened. She helped me pick out my first bra.

"She was gentle, but later I learned she was made of steel. She came for a long period when Mother was dying; she was a lot like your mom. I was sixteen; my father and I were just about stressed out. Right away she relieved me of cooking and keeping track of my mother's medications. She suggested we call hospice, and her presence made all the difference. Ellie, I miss the both of them so much.

"But, what I wanted to say is that like my aunt, there's softness to your mother's face that even losing Da hasn't taken away. But Ellie, inside she's strong. Ellie, you're so like her. You and I don't have that extended time away from each other, but I guess if we did I would write my heart to you. I love you, Ellie, and I've only said it once all evening."

"I love you too. For me, reading these is a door to my mother's heart. I think by allowing us to read them, she's saying two things: She has accepted you as my partner, and she's asking me to step into a closeness that we've not had in the past. She and Da were so intense about loving each other. Something about their letters gives me even more freedom to be myself, something I've been reluctant about for so long. I was afraid to talk about my needs. Who wants to disappoint their mom?"

"You're right. It's only natural to want people to understand, especially something as important as your sexuality. Few daughters ever know their mother like that. I feel as if she's given us her blessing to be a couple."

"She needs you to know her and she wants to know and understand you. I can tell that meeting me is really important to her. Shall we read until we're through?" Maddy says.

"Yes, let's do. It seems a miracle that we're here in Belle Haven where they used to meet and forget the rest of the world. When we lived in Santa Cruz, sometimes she would go to painting workshops or on business trips about Mr. Sari's property. I never asked where she went. I was in the band, and we played every weekend. Sonya and I were together a lot of the time. I loved Sonya's mom. I loved Sonja. I was always welcome. She never chided us when we got home a little late. That's when I tried my first cigarette. I'm sure she smelled it!"

Ellie picks up another letter, checking to see if the dates are in order.

December 3, 1982
Washington

> Suze, my constant companion and Love,
>
> To keep a low profile, I am writing this as if I am writing a report so my nosy secretary won't catch on immediately. Already, she gets overexcited when you call and is dying to know all about you.

A SEASON OF MISTS

I returned to work on the third and have faithfully trotted off to the post office at lunchtime, on each of the last three days. Each time the empty box reminded me of a coffin, prepared for a funeral – an omen? No, I cannot believe that our mutual love is suddenly doomed to cease, pass out of existence or evaporate. I simply cannot believe or accept that because I believe in your love for me, while my own life for the last two years has been governed and motivated by my love for you.

Nevertheless, I am human, and I am gifted with an enormous imagination which has grown and waxed after many years of experience. If I haven't heard, is it because of a lessening of love on either side? What is it then? Are you ill? Has something happened in your family, preventing you from sending me even the smallest letter or card, at least? Have you had a change of mind, or did you make a New Year's resolution to make the supreme sacrifice and kill all thoughts of me? Why, why, why do I not hear a single word from you? With each day, my worries grow, and depression takes a firmer hold on me.

Oh, Suze, if you only knew how constantly you are in my thoughts; how I talk to you from hour to hour, as if you are there, at my side; how the longing for you never, never subsides, instead grows and grows until it becomes almost unbearable; yes, how I love you, deeply, purely as well as passionately at all times of day and night regardless of seasons, or weather, or up and down moods… always.

Yes, I fully realize that I owe you a long, long letter, especially after the heartrending, beautiful, sensitive letter you wrote when visiting your dying aunt. (Were you able to go to the funeral?) That was, and is such a beautiful letter, that each time I read it, tears come to my eyes; and the desire to hold you in my arms, just hold you and comfort you, become so enormous that I wonder how I can ever go on living without you!

Thursday

Now I am beginning to wonder whether you actually received my last, very hastily written and brief letter with a picture of me in Paraguay where I stayed in an old Jesuit Mission. Paraguay is considered the *Corazón de América* ("Heart of America"). The Gurani culture continues to thrive, and I speak neither that nor much of the heavily accented Spanish. Are you interested in these details, my darling, which fascinate me? I'll be glad to spend some time with family. I dashed the letter off, one hour before we left Washington on vacation to Idaho.

Soon, with artificial hearts, (what a coup) we can all live forever…

All my love,

Da

12 December 1982
Miami Airport

My Love, my lover, my Suze

You may be disappointed when you receive this letter, for ninety-nine percent of it is written by yourself. As usual, I am carrying your letters with me, wherever I go, not just because I cherish them, but I find it increasingly risky to leave them behind.

It also tears me apart, if I were to start tearing them up again. Your letters are just too beautiful and precious to end up in a waste basket or for someone else to read them. So, I'll take your suggestion and embrace the idea. Why not start a book together? You apparently keep my letters. Perhaps, combined, they may inspire some wandering souls in this world someday. Do you want to handle it this way? What it amounts to, is that I give the sole copyright of everything I have ever written to you, and hopefully will write to you. Do with it what you want only do a lot of editing of names and all.

You will also note that I have made some annotations in your letters to save time and to react immediately to some of your more urgent observations.

This was one of those missions again. Work, work, work and dashing from one place to another, never alone and never a moment's rest! I thought of you constantly and talked to you, day and night.

Our brief encounter in L.A. did leave me with a warm inner glow, a peaceful state of mind, which I did not know I was able to experience again. Thinking of you made me feel whole, satisfied, happy, serenely happy but also with a deep nostalgia for your eyes and lips, and warm, soft body. I love you, my dearest darling.

I wanted to write you so badly but just never found the time. Last night in the plane, I was in the usual state of euphoria when I have a few hours of rest ahead of me but instead of writing you I fell asleep – conked out. I was just too exhausted and didn't wake up until close to landing. Now, I'll be on my way to Washington in a few minutes.

In the meantime, thank you again, my lover for being you, for going through all sorts of traumatic difficulties to meet me at the drop of a hat. I do appreciate that more than I can say or express. You're putting a lot of miles on that car of yours. Are you getting mileage from the airlines for your flights?

I love you so much I feel like bursting.
Forever yours, Da

(Cont'd)
12/22/82

That was a crazy day. All along I had been planning to write you in the one week between my return from South America and our departure from Washington but there was simply no time. I had sleepless nights, and if, by chance I did sleep, I had nightmares. Finally, on that Monday morning before taking off, I saw a chance to write you a few lines. I had to take the dog to the kennel and have the car washed. I wrote the note in the car wash!

In a way, I was also rather upset by your beautiful and moving letter. Somehow, I had a feeling that you were blaming me for nourishing a very passionate and strictly physical love for you to make myself feel young again; to enjoy the excitement of just an affair. So, let me reiterate: I love you. I love you wholly – I love You, for who and what you are, for your sensitivity, thoughtfulness, compassion, empathy, your sense of duty, devotion, charity, intelligence, appreciation of life – everything. I also love you because you love me; and yes, I love your body, too. I love your fine face, your soft eyes, your young figure, the warm welcome of your womanly embrace. I love all of you; and in the brief times we share together, I try to enjoy it all: your company, you talking and listening, your eyes darting in the same direction as mine, your ears tuned in to the same sounds as mine, our togetherness, our mutual adoration and joint appreciation, and I would not be human if I did not enjoy our love-making as well.

When I think of you, as I do constantly, I do not think of you naked and stretched out ready to receive me. Sure, I do now and then, sometimes perhaps more than not, but not primarily so. I think of you as a constant companion, sitting by my side, in the office, in meetings, in my car, while commuting, walking together in the woods, swimming together in the ocean, side by side in the movies, theater or concert hall, shopping together for clothes and jewels for you. Yes, just living together and enjoying each other's company.

Of course, every day ends eventually, and I see us together again at last on a balcony or porch overlooking the Mediterranean or an Alpine valley, or in front of the fireplace at Belle Haven, listening to Brahms or Mahler, leafing through art books, sipping wine, eating crackers and cheese or pâté. Finally, getting ready for bed with anticipation and desire building up the nearer we get to the bedroom suite, and the final voluptuous move into bed, between soft and warm sheets, rolling over towards each other, embracing each other with arms and legs entwined in such a way, that each knows we can depend on each other. Just holding each other, softly but firmly, feeling the other's heartbeat and breath, hands and fingers caressing, feeling oh, so happy and content to be... just together.

When?

Ever?

Friday

I find that writing you has an appeasing influence on my somber and dark mood. At least, I am talking to you directly this way, and somehow, I imagine you listening to me and responding.

Coming back from the post office today, the fifth unsuccessful search in a row this week, I decided that I should not really expect frequent, long letters from you. I know how busy you are, and how much is at stake for you to do this job right. I am sure everyone is making demands on you without any letup. Also, and that was really the most important conclusion I reached: after having received your last letter, what more can I expect? If anything, you made it patently clear that you love me and that your love is of exceptional magnitude and quality – I agree – but in your desperation and frustration, you said I might tend to shape you into my dream image of you, therewith threatening my sense of you retaining your own identity.

I suffer frustration and shudder when I think of a future without you. Yet, I cannot give you up. I love you too dearly for that. I suffer while I revel in the beauty of our love; I agonize while being in ecstasy. My heart hurts all over, while my flesh tingles in anticipation of our bodily contact and, yet I'd rather have it this way than not have your love.

Your Da

Maddy, stands and stretches. "May I bring you something El'?"
"Let's have tea," Ellie says.
"Maddy, I didn't know it was like this for her. Through her pain and through her dream of what could be, she didn't hear him when he said he wouldn't leave Cora. She just couldn't bear to hear it."
"I think by leasing Belle Haven, he gave her even more hope. So torn himself, he took a huge step to find a place she would fall in love with. And he knew her roots were here in the northwest, that she loved the sea." Maddy chuckles, "I think she fell in love with this place almost as hard as she had for him. It became home in her mind. He had to have known it would persuade her to continue seeing him. Look how they have expressed themselves throughout."
"How we all long to make a home. I guess I didn't realize it quite so much until we met." Ellie says
They sip the tea, an Earl Grey, holding it with both hands, blowing away the steam.
"I can see that what he sees and hears from her touched him in the deepest of places. No wonder he returned and returned. Ellie, I see her differently than

you can as her daughter. I think her letters to him reflect how she was searching. She wanted love not to be a myth. She was willing to pay a high price to keep that as a truth for her. They both did. They felt they had found the something more, the unfabled, that something everyone seeks."

It is Maddy's voice again as they pick up from where they left off.

February 1, 1983

> My love, I am propped up by pillows, sleepy, still warm from my bath, thinking of you – you must tire of this scene – as you go off again on another journey without me. I'm dazzled by your life, envious a little I guess. I'm hungry for your touch, your voice. The shadow of your presence always plays on the periphery of my thinking; I reach out for you, and while recall brings you into the embrace of my thoughts, a longing I am never sure whether to welcome or reject fills me up. The choice doesn't matter because the longing is inevitable, something I don't get to choose against. It remains no matter how I steer my way. It is nearly the thirteenth anniversary of our meeting. I wonder about the passing of time and the redemption of it for us, for our love.
>
> Sunday, beautifully clear and crisp, found me far down the beach climbing over debris from the storm. I climbed out on the jetty and sat perched overlooking the yacht harbor, and with the ocean air in my face, the clanging of the bells, the squeaks of the rubber tires against the vessels, I pulled you again into these kind of moments we've spent apart but which I've associated with you as the deepest part of me calls to you, crying for a miracle.
>
> Time (the best of times) goes unredeemed. Our best years are here and now. Already, my heart leaps ahead to mid-'83, and if our meeting doesn't take place I'll leap ahead to the next date you give me.

Your letters are no substitute, but they are a taste of our future as I guzzle up your expressions of love for me, waiting for the next offering.

Your Suze

February 1, 1983

My darling,

To think you won't receive this until you return March 4. Time has always played a rascal role in our relationship, also a mysterious one, the passing of it; ignored as if we believe in the hereafter and plan to spend it together. You seemed to have found your niche, and I am still flailing about trying to discover mine, and now at post mid-life am baffled by my struggle.

I know you know as I map out my way that I have to leave a road open to you — I just must. Suze, I would love to have a child together. Dare we even think of it?

I have deliberately chosen this notebook paper so I can write without a great degree of filtering… more later.

Da

March 27, 1983

My dearest Da,

How often through these years I've come to you and written my heart to you and always with the sweet assurance you heard me and loved me. Now, these past most painful weeks

I haven't been able to pen anything to you... some deep resentment about you being away, that you are so far from me and always will be has welled up and forced closed those doors that always opened so readily to you.

To think that you love me as you do, and yet, you wait; I wait, just as in my marriage I was always waiting. I have come to the conclusion I shan't make that choice, to not be the primary person in someone's life and yet your voice, your letters, your bared soul cause me to throw away the most practical ideas about how to live my life. My God, Da, I've needed you now. My pain isn't the result of a selfish fling. This pain is a result of trying to be true to myself because I can no longer justify my existence unless I succeed in being my own person. I'm plenty scared and don't think you have stopped to either imagine my fears or realize how realistically founded they are.

Oh, yes, the sometimes would-be suitors, but who are they? Perfume, flowers, is not where I am. (I do like the perfume you've given me. The roses were lovely too. I'm fickle, I suppose.) I treasure everything you've given me, especially the unbroken braid of gold I wear daily, but I question everything when I look at it.

I've got a life to hack out of some pretty stubborn soil, because I've been so entrenched in this fundamental subculture that I now see as more unfertile than I realized. Has an education "of sorts" fouled my ability to be founded in Christ? My father always said I was the child of the King. But that would make for a lot of princesses, wouldn't it?

So life opens up to me little by little, sometimes in surges, strong and vibrant, sometimes in a flood of unexpected tears. I'm not always crying, believe me. But I'm alive again to my own inner direction, the signals internal and insistent.

Always now, when I embrace thoughts of you I sense the peril of waiting. You know or you don't that if I can't be primary in your life as you lead it and make choices, I have to give myself the gift of letting you go. Belle Haven or no, it is so hard. I can't be content otherwise. That you give yourself to another while you cry for me. I understand your inability to leave all and come to me... then everyone experiences pain. I understand that she is afraid, how it persists from the dark years in the Netherlands, even though here in America her fears of being persecuted as a Jew are unfounded. The point is the fact that I've loved you so long is causing additional pain right now and steals from me my ability to love anyone else. I feel burnt out, as if I have given all there is to give to two men, and it has moved neither to be my companion. In spirit, yes, but I believe you cannot be my companion ever... really. I'm seeing Michael.

I feel bitterness. The strength of my passion has been played out like the surf against the rocks, wasted energy, however beautiful. To what avail, those races up I-680 to see you when you were still in Sacramento, the readiness now to run to you in Washington, or Belle Haven, the endless hours I have conversed with you in my heart? To what avail to be alone in the time of greatest need, to have you so far away, always so damn far from me. God, I'm a fool. You know my heart, always so exposed and naked to you.

I want to make my own way and never love with total abandon again. That's where I am. No, to Hawaii. No, to waiting until May. I've every day to face without hope of any return on my investment of thirteen years. To be sought after seems meaningless, and I've no heart for it... not the lovemaking or the high drama of the dreaded last moments when we say good-bye. You speak of me as being your constant companion, but I've not been. I only see the contrails. I've been here while you take wing, while you are in the slipstream. You bring me into a pretend world, even to the extent of suggesting a baby.

Oh, God Da, go to hell and let me be.

Love forever,

Suze

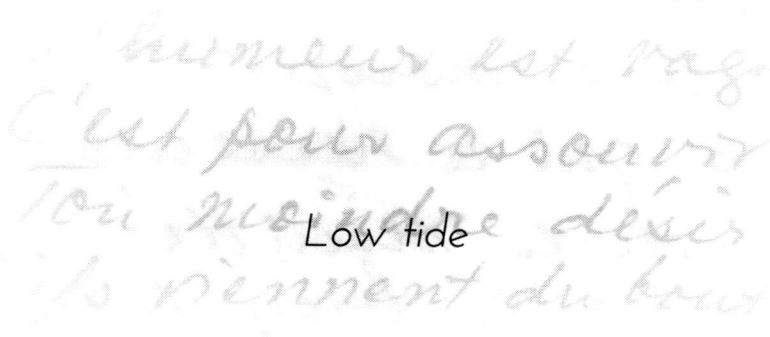

Low tide

1 April, 1983

> I am sending this letter back to you. I have made notes and comments in the margins.
>
> I made those to emphasize points I want to discuss with you in my return letters.
>
> One thing comes out very clearly in this whole series-overtime: no matter what happened, and in spite of the misery and strain you've had to live with... you love me... and for that I am so grateful.
>
> Words from my side cannot begin to express the emotions I undergo when I read your letters and sense that enormous love you pour into them.
>
> You are all *woman*! My woman!
>
> Yours, Da

Ellie has stretched out with her head in Maddy's lap.

"I can't believe he sends the letter right back to her, saying it is an avowal of her love for him," Ellie says.

"Ellie, neither of them accept the fact they won't have some life together. They agonize. Their obsession is unbelievable!"

"But look what they got. They did get these years together. I understand their feelings. I waited so long for you to come along. I knew there was someone. Now, I couldn't let you go, no matter the obstacles, even if you had another partner."

1 April 1983

My dearest Suze,

Good Friday and a hint of spring in the air. The magnolias are in full bloom on Pennsylvania Avenue, in front of our bank building. The sky is clear, the cold wind has finally died down; thank God, spring is coming. I always feel marvelous this time of the year, the combination of Easter and spring; the promise of new life, new ideas, new ambitions, bright thoughts.

But, somehow, I am sad and depressed. I feel let down and I am disappointed, oh so disappointed. I keep wondering, "Why doesn't she write me anymore?" And, then, your letter…

That question has become an obsession and a nightmare, because after our call, last Saturday, I really thought you were going to write me. Then again, watching *The Thorn Birds*, I was convinced that you would write, assuming you were watching it too, and would be struck by the overwhelming similarities in the lives of Meggie and Ralph and you and me.

But nothing came from your side. In desperation, I spent half an hour in church yesterday and again today (between the Easter services. I hate crowded churches, and I love to be in one, almost deserted so I can feel His presence all to myself). I prayed for you, and I prayed for enlightenment, that I would understand.

And, I guess He heard me and made me understand you are relishing your new-won freedom and have decided it should be a total freedom, a total abandonment of old ties, with a husband who would not understand your needs, and with a lover who wanted to possess you, but could give nothing in return.

I cannot blame you. As Ralph, the priest in *The Thorn Birds* says, "I know I have hurt you deeply all my life, but I want you to know, I have loved you, oh so much."

Suze, my dearest Suze, if you want to free yourself of me, do so. It is your life, not mine; you should be free at this crucial point in your life, to make your own decisions and not to get confused by a lover who is tugging on your heart.

I know I have been naïve and selfish to think that you would waste your thoughts, dreams and desires on me, now that you are free. Forgive me, my Love.

Oh, how I love you. True, I would like to be with you now, more than ever to help you make your decisions, etc. Who do I think I am? Just as well, then, that I am not with you. Yes, it's very presumptuous of me to think that you need me now, now of all times!

Again, forgive me but I am only human, and I did not doubt for one moment your love for me.

You will have new vistas and new ideas – wonderful! I should rejoice with you and perhaps with some effort, I will. It's just that I am too bloody human. In your new life, that you recently started, you must have found me too possessive, and too much in love with you. Now it hurts to see you leave me, to go your own way, to live without my love, without my mental support but that's, after all, as it should be.

You must manage alone, for that's the road you have chosen now, at least for the time being. Once you can stand squarely on your own domain, and are sure that this is the life you want, you can afford to reach out again and indulge in loving and being loved, I hope you will then remember me and call on me, if you ever feel the urge or the need. For my dearest, dearest Suze, you are my love, my constant companion, my muse, the personification of all that is humanly good, true and beautiful, of youth, eternal youth and freshness, and above all: a truly lovely young woman – my soul-mate!

I love you Suze, and I shall never stop loving you but I don't want to stand in your way, in the way of your own life's fulfillment.

I repeat from that beautiful, beautiful card you sent the other day:

> *What I can offer is simply me. All I can ask*
> *Is for you to be honest and open.*

Please, please, my darling, whatever you decide, be honest, and let me know whether or not I still play a role in your life.

It is your decision, your will, your life and I will understand.

Right now, I am sad, not only because I am on the verge of losing you, but because you would not let me know how you felt about these things going through your mind.

(You were definitely different over the phone, last week; Saturday, I could sense your change of mind!)

To top off my sadness and depression this week, I got word from Hawaii yesterday, that they had cancelled the conference in May.

So that's out, too.

Maybe just as well?

I love you Suze

Your Da

MYRNA BROWN

(Old stationery from my business in California)
April 16, 1983

My dearest Suze,

See how thrifty I am, I still have paper from our California days.

I am sitting here in the County Library, not far from where we live, taking my refuge on a Saturday afternoon, for I simply must write you.

When I returned home from work last night, I was very depressed. All week long, I'd wanted to write you, but I just got around to it, because the report I'm working on (Cameroon's Palm Nut Oil Project) kept me busy. Each time I thought I had it finished, another item cropped up, which I felt I still ought to cover in greater detail and there went another day of painstaking research.

It is true that life filled to its full Kodachrome glory, after I talked with you over the phone about a week ago, a few days after I received that dismal letter of yours. You cannot imagine how desperately sad I felt after reading that letter. On the one hand, I had more or less anticipated it and could wholeheartedly agree with you (which I indicated in my own letter which crossed yours). But then, the force of your anguished words struck me right where it hurt most: my ego, my pedantic notion that I had been good to you at least in a small way, that I had helped you through my listening and reacting, at least to some extent, had helped you find yourself and your own way. Yes, I was deeply hurt, and all color flowed out of my life, then and there.

In a way, I felt there was nothing to look forward to anymore. What was the use to continue this work, if it isn't in the hope to get to Belle Haven or pass through S.F. and L.A. anymore to see you, my darling. Why continue to commute back and forth to work, bathing my ears with romantic music, so I can dream of you while driving? Why bother if she wants me to go to hell, and forget me forever?

I remember vividly, the next morning (after receiving your letter) I had not slept a wink that night and when I got up, the sky was gray, it rained, everything was wet, and the world presented itself to me in all shades of gray and black, and I thought, "What the hell, there's no hope for tender love and adventure at Suze's side anymore. There is no future of laughter, emotion, ecstasy and agony, just this dull humdrum life: the nagging at home, the conniving at the office, the suspicion of government officials in the countries where I work, the endless travel, the bleak hotel rooms. Blah, I might as well quit and pack my bags and roam the world, become a beachcomber in the hope that someday, someday, many years from now I will meet you again. I have never felt so miserable in my life. Oh, I do love you so much Suze. You have no idea. And, yes, I am so unrealistic about it, too. Perhaps it is the reaction of having to be 100 percent realistic, at all times, when at work. Bankers and moneylenders do not believe in dreams and "ifs". So, let me be, let me dream, let me live in my own nirvana, in my after-working hours. Then I can dream of you and scheme, and hope, and pray, and let my heart sing out for you.

Perhaps it is not fair to you and if it means you suffer by it, then you must cut me out of your life for good. Somehow, I keep thinking and hoping it may affect you in the same fashion as it does me. At least we have the certainty and consolation of each other's love — that is something real and something to hold on to. Love conquers all according to St. Paul and I firmly believe that. It may hurt, yes, I may hurt like hell but still there's love —something beautiful and undefinable. For how many poets and authors have not tried to describe love, finding that it takes a whole lot of words to describe only its qualities or symptoms, or effects? But what is love — the stuff people will suffer for all their lives, for which most, will gladly give their life, their future, their very existence!

So love is there, and that's about all we share! Love can make us strong, and help move mountains, if need be. Love can help us persevere and keep struggling to reach the goal we've set for ourselves. Love endures everything: pain and solitude, and absence. On the other hand, with love, our life's quality is enhanced; it lends greatness and beauty to our lives and, if and when we finally meet again, love is there to turn our joy to rapture, our happiness to ecstasy, our dreams to outbursts of creativity, our songs to oratorios, and our mere existences to glorious living

I suppose it is the briefness of our meetings which makes it so, for no human soul could endure such intensity of love and life for too long. I want to try! That's why I see our rare (and I admit all too brief) get-togethers as not only essential, but life-giving to such an extent that we may nourish our soul, and achieve fulfillment, which will make us go forth again for some time to come.

If you can see it in that vein too, I shall be very happy.

And if you agree, I shall again try everything in my power to have us meet again soon. Tomorrow, come our first guests from Kenya; followed by a daughter, then my brother, Jaan; then another daughter. We'll be free, finally, by mid-May. If I cannot make it to Belle Haven you'd better come here. I would love to see you here and show you around this fair city. All my love, my very dearest.

Embraces and kisses, yours forever,

Da

A SEASON OF MISTS

May 27, 1983

My dearest Love,

Another week shot again. I spent it on doing some spring cleaning in my office, getting my files in order, etc. etc. A luxury I have not been able to afford myself since I joined the organization.

So, as you see I'm not very busy, and getting awfully restless — ready to go on a mission.

And how have you been yourself, my dearest Suze? I keep thinking of you and how you are and on the other hand, somewhat sad or how exciting, and exhilarating your life must be these days. But, I am convinced that with your newly-won independence and freedom and faith in yourself, you will be able to cope. Yes, I am sure you will succeed now that you have made your first big step. I will be with you in thoughts and prayers. Yes, I want you to succeed and lead your own life as you see fit…

(British Airways Concourse paper)

You can do it and I will gladly step aside and remove myself as a possible hurdle in this already arduous path you have chosen. Gladly? No not really, i.e., not gladly from my side, but glad to do it for you, if it helps you.

Already, I have begun to resign myself to a future without you; a very bleak future, indeed. But I must think in this direction, for I must leave you totally free; any personal interjection or appearance or effort from my side, will most likely construe to be an interference in your progress on the path of freedom. Going through a divorce is no sinecure. I have personally witnessed the misery and confusion my secretary went through for the last two to three years. It will be a period of heartbreak and resignation for you but something you feel you must do, because there is a promise of a better life, beyond all this. Thus, you will sway between despair and hope, between grief and joy but you will carry on and fight; and fight because you want to succeed.

And, once it is all behind you, and you have gained your freedom, you'll have another difficult and thorny path to go. May it be brief and more rosy than thorny but once more you will have to grit your teeth together to force yourself to make the ultimate right choice – your choice. What are you going to do next with your life? Are you going to be career woman, truly liberated, free and proud and self-sufficient; choosing your own friends and companions on your terms and when you feel like it? Or are you going to succumb to promises of love and leisure, by a well-meaning, loving individual, who will promise and offer wealth and comfort as long as you marry him? Either way may turn out to be the ideal situation (especially if the man, whoever he is, is honest and capable of following up). Either way can also turn out to be disastrous. You want to be sure to make the right choice, then and there. I know, I am redundant.

Whatever you do, or decide, or choose, I am afraid I will be in your way, because my presence or utterances may just color or deflect your intentions or decisions.

Don't get me wrong, I would love to be involved deeply and intimately in your life and your decisions but, I love you so much and desire you so passionately that I cannot trust myself to give you the appropriate advice, or any guidance at all! I am only too human, my dear, dear Suze, and anything I do or say might just be inspired by purely selfish motives. Because in the final analysis, I want you and I would want you all to myself.

I am going crazy thinking about you, and dreaming about how I would love you and treat you and spoil you, if you were mine. Time and again, I make shopping trips with you, draping you in the finest dresses, hanging luminous jewelry around your neck, until you are radiant from the glamour of it all. (Your simplicity is your beauty; don't let me change that about you.) And, I travel with you, taking you to my favorite places and hideouts and seeking forever new ones.

I cannot stop loving you Suze, at least not now, not ever, I think. But I must leave you free and if you ever decide to be totally free, or if you suddenly do remarry, and find your chosen Prince I'll slink away and disappear out of your life willingly, i.e. out of my own willpower, but not without pain and agony, in the realization that I will then lose you forever.

Time will tell. In the meantime, I'll try to write you now and then, assuming, somewhat vainly, that you do want to hear from me.

If not, please drop me a line to that effect, and I shall stop.

I love you Suze, now more than ever. Both my heart and flesh are crying out for you. Yes, darling, I miss you terribly.

Do take care, my Love…

Forever your Da

Morning mists

Bogota
May 1983

My dearest love,

Just a note to let you know you are still constantly in my thoughts. Not a day, not an hour passes without thinking of you. If you only knew how terribly I miss you and how depressed I become when I cannot find any chance of arranging some immediate get-together again. The situation is very bleak; suddenly the pipeline of projects seems to have dried up. The only vague possibility of a mission is an appraisal in Kenya, (more coffee) which lies east of here, not west. Perhaps I can arrange a series of supervision missions to South America, and make a slight detour to the west coast. Still and all, it won't be until July, now that I can finally break away from here. My annual leave has now been fixed for June – about the tenth to the thirtieth.

Enough of that "keep hoping" I tell myself. There will come a time – let's hope you still want to see me then!

Suze, my loveliest, my real lover (yes, you are so real in my thoughts and dreams). I keep looking at you, and see all the details of your sweet face, your little nose, your earlobes, your smile, your lips, your eyes. Oh, yes, you are real and not just a dream.

A SEASON OF MISTS

Suze, I am so terribly proud of you for having achieved what you recently did. First of all, for landing yourself a very good and very demanding and responsible job with all the benefits. Good-bye and good luck to that bastard Indian. And, now your master coup of doubling your salary. I am very, very proud of you. You're a writer, albeit a technical writer of 'Secret' documents. You can work yourself up the ladder now. Congratulations! I hate that your commute is so long, clear over to San Jose. It's a challenge to drive those curves.

I hope also that this (your achievement) has sufficiently bolstered your ego to wipe out, once and for all, all vague and half-hearted feelings of inadequacy or inferiority into the trash can! You are magnificent!

I am proud to know you and have your love. I do believe, I still believe, that you love me and so do I love you forever, until death does us part.

I only wish you could be mine.

I love you so much Suze, really and truly. I find life unbearable without you. I find it tedious and dull and unexciting now and only live for the day that I shall hold you in my arms again. Oh, Love, love, love, how painful is your sting…

Da

Miami airport – Bogota
July 24, 1983

My dearest Love,

First, I wanted to call you this morning before leaving for S.F., but it was too early. Then I thought of doing it from here but this departure lounge in an apparent new wing in this airport is known for its non-accommodations: no telephone, no air conditioning, and 95°F. About 97.5 percent of the passengers are agitated Latinos! On top of that, our connecting flight to Bogota is delayed by at least two hours! Hurrah, for travelling during summer vacation time! (It took twenty minutes alone to get through the security check line, not that they did anything special, but the number of passengers was just too great to handle.)

Otherwise, no news whatsoever and that's the idea. I love you and you love me deeply and tenderly and each contact, be it note, a visit, a touch, a look, a word of love, or a mutual appreciation of Brahms sends me into ecstasy and utter delight, while simultaneously sending warnings of agonizing tremors. Yet, we accept it willingly, because we are not prepared, at least, not yet, to close the door on each other. Are you really back?

Give us another little while, dear God, to digest and savor the goodness and beauty of our mutual love. With time, we may eventually settle for reality, demanding a gradual loosening of our physical ties, while perhaps holding on forever to pure and all-encompassing love, on a more platonic level.

Let's not let it worry us now. No need to stare ourselves blind on that event before the time comes. All in all, I hope your enjoyment of this last get-together (last = most recent, not necessarily last last!) was as great as mine. In spite of the tears and the pain it brought, too! I had worked myself up to such a miserable frenzy and state of deep depression that I could not find any plausible, reasonable and happy solution any more before my coming.

And there, suddenly, the good Lord answered my fervent prayers and we did meet again, as before, and even more so; more secure, more relaxed, happier, and more meaningful. It was all there and it was great beyond description! I love you, my darling Suze. Thank you, my love, for being yourself, through and through. Be good, take care, and all my love. Now, next I can look forward to seeing you again there where you've made your little home in Santa Cruz. Keeping the children in their same schools is important. Rather than give up that little spot of paradise, I'm glad you've decided to commute. Do you like the RX7?

Forever, your Da

P.S. You say you'll be up for promotion soon to the next grade. You'll be a GS-12!

P.S.S. Remind me. I must commend Frank and the housekeeper. Belle Haven looked so fine and ready for us. Frank lays a good fire. But, without you, were I there, I would be wretched. It is a place too beautiful in which to be alone.

July 27, 1983

My dearest Da,

It's Wednesday, an eternity since you left. I feel as if I have just left a sick bed, physically weak, emotionally near tears or actually in tears, unexpectedly. I can't seem to adjust to you having been in this room and now gone.

I've left to me the business of living, of making decisions, even what I eat, talking while my mind reverts over and over again to the slightest of reminders of our time here.

I feel so very weary, spent, yet so tender and sensitive. I want that refuge of who we are together, yet I want to be aware of reality and all that's being required of me. I know that I love you more. I can't bear not seeing you for a long time. But if I saw you often, and didn't have you solely for myself, it would be hell indeed. I'm going to work my way to you. Maybe a transfer.

I don't want to love you. My tired mind and heart seek the refuge of simplicity, of the mundane, the practical, of the savior that routine can be. I thought I had desensitized myself to want you, but desire swells and heaves as a child being born. As I was for each child, I am afraid of the responsibility that comes with physically holding you. You've tracked me through that underbrush my life has been, kept me in your heart.

We must promise ourselves to spare each other, not to ever again experience rejection or fear of rejection. I had stopped believing you, and I colored your motives. I read your letters in a slanted way. Today, now, I believe you again. Nothing will take it away, even if you leave me one day.

Everything is in terms of you, the Rachmaninoff, the morning fog, the roses, still so stately in their vase, my rumpled bed where you came to me. Oh, the scent of you, barely a scent...

All the details of life — seeing the lawyer (I'm not asking for support because David wssn't paid well and has lost his job because I've left him) — but also, beautiful moments when the sun finally pierces the dense Monterey Bay fog. You are with me all the time. I'm talking with you, looking to you, or being strong or compassionate because of you. It's a reflection of what you've often expressed, that we have a presence with each other that is not physical.

Don't let's loosen these ties that hold us together. I want to experience you in every way I may. When I was a girl, I believed this kind of love existed. I have to believe this love is real.

I must go

love, forever.

Suze

A SEASON OF MISTS

Peru
July 27, 1983

My very dearest Suze,

At last a brief moment of rest. I'm having dinner by myself in one of those antique Spanish restaurants thinking of you, luxuriating in *dolce-far-niente,* after a very hectic and busy week of meeting, conferences, promotion talks, etc.

I want you to know my Love, my Angel that an indescribable peace has descended upon me, at last. During the day, in spite of the compressed work schedule, I can smile again and find myself laughing heartily. At night, *Mon Dieu,* I can sleep again, uninterruptedly for at least six hours. A far, far cry from the nervous breakdown I had during the last three to four months, worried about you. (I'm writing this on the back of an appointment slip from Banco Nacional de la Sabena.)

July 29, 1983

Last night during dinner (alone), I started to write you on the only slip of paper I could find in my pocket. Tonight, I came better prepared, although the size of the paper is not much greater.

After arriving in Lima today at about 1 p.m., I went out for a long walk (4.5 hours!) and thought of you all during that walk, talking to you as if you were strolling beside me. So now I must write again to record my thoughts of today.

As I said (wrote), I am in a most euphoric state of mind after our get together last week. The contrast of how I felt before is unbelievable. You probably know how miserable I felt judging from my behavior in the car, after our dinner at La Chaumière. The unhappiness of the previous months had built up to such a pitch, that I simply could not control myself after seeing you again. I hope you will forgive me my very unmanly behavior. In spite of how I nearly attacked you, you returned my affections with like passion.

Now, that has all changed. Seeing you again, and seeing how you have matured during this last year, made me very, very happy because to me it was proof of your right decision. You simply would not be what you are now, had you not made that fateful decision in January of '82. After hearing about your life, over the many ups and downs of your marital status, I can only admire you for having stuck it out that long, against all odds, and in the face of no improvement, even with the counselling.

You deserve better! That is for sure. You asked me why I love you. Do I need to answer after all that? It is simply because you are the purest-loving, most honest, most sacrificing, most noble woman I know. And besides, you are beautiful – you have a lovely ingratiating face (and a beautiful, warm, soft, huggable body!), and the most charming way of meeting the people and world around you. You are also very observant and get turned on by the same wonderful things in nature and life as I do. You love the singing of the birds in the morning and the full-bodied sounds of orchestral music, composed by the classical greats.

I could go on and on singing your praises…

But to get back to my visit. I was overjoyed to see how your looks and smiles had gained a new luster and a most endearing appeal of depth and maturity – born of suffering, no doubt – but also out of appreciation of having embraced a new, more independent lifestyle.

You are so utterly gorgeous that I find it difficult not to be in constant physical touch with you when we are together.

A SEASON OF MISTS

And yet, strangely enough, in spite of the intense longing I have for you, I am at ease and can live in peace with myself and the consequences of loving you.

Why?

Probably because I am now wholly convinced that you will continue to love me as I do you. I know you have fought with the decision to close the door on me, and at the same time you have fought with the decision to continue our love-tryst. Your most inner feelings and wisdom have won and in your heart you have considered that come what may, whether you will marry again or not, you will always love me and so will I. I will always love you, darling, until death does us part.

The mango you brought me after our lovemaking, dipping my spoon into its chilled, ripe flesh was heaven, like you, my darling.

Da

The ebb and flow

Paraguay
August 3, 1983

My Suze,

I so hoped to be able to write you again while here but my days and evenings continue to be too busy. In Paraguay (where I arrived Saturday night very late), I have been to the home of the local project manager of our project, a most charming Portuguese gentleman with an interesting genealogical background about which he is all too eager to tell you, when he knows you well enough. His thirty-six-year-old (second) wife – he is fifty-two – is also highly intelligent, but if anything, I am just plain worried about her, because she has all sorts of ailments and most of the time she looks sick.

I had a quiet Sunday, talking business and generalities with him and on Monday we flew a single engine Cessna to the hacienda to supervise the project.

During the day, I began to feel more and more miserable, because it was bloody cold and I was not dressed for it. On our way back however, I began to feel very feverish and by the time we got home I was shaking like a reed, had indeed a high fever, felt alternately very cold and very hot. By midnight, I felt like dying but after several quinine pills and about ten aspirins, the fever finally subsided by early morning leaving me feel like a wrung-out dishrag. Lo, and behold, I have spent most of my life in the tropics and here I had finally my first bout of malaria (I must have picked it up in Columbia).

Today, three days later, I feel okay, thanks to loads of quinine and aspirin.

Let's get back to my little notes. It is because I am convinced now that you still love me and will keep on loving me as I do you that I can maintain that heavenly peace within me. I also believe our brief get together, in a serenely, quiet environment – your own home – deepened the love for each other and, whenever we have for each other and whenever we shall meet again that will repeat itself. We shall continue to grow in love and we shall reach the most sublime level of loving, eventually a love totally void of guilt feelings. On the contrary, a love so great and devoted that everything will pale in its shine and radiance.

Oh, my lovely Suze, I love you so much, and I am so grateful to you for being yourself and for having had the courage to receive me again at home, and within your own self. Oh, glorious, wonderful, all-encompassing love. Oh, delicious nectar of passion, ardor, and devotion, of being able to let one's self flow into the other – to become one in ecstasy.

I love you so much darling, I can yell, shout and sing and jubilate, so the whole world will know I love you.

Life has taken on a new, fresh dimension for me. There is *you* again, as the focus of my thinking, drawing tremendous centripetal force for my thoughts and desires.

Yes, I do long for you, I do desire and lust for you and yet, and this is a totally new phenomenon in me. I don't let the present unfulfilled desire be a frustration (I sense now your commitment to me). Instead, the desire now works positively in that it creates a new hope for a new meeting, another and greater intensification of pure love.

Come to me in your dreams, my Love, and tell me that I am not dreaming, that I am right.

I shall mail this in San Paulo where I will be tomorrow. I hope it will reach you.

I also hope that I may find a letter from you, or at least an acknowledgment, of having received this.

You have made me strong and loving... I can stand a lot now, but I still would like to hear from you now and then, to drag me away from the pit of despair, which inevitably opens up at my feet, when total silence (from your side) takes over.

Please don't let that happen, I just cannot face another crisis like that again. I love you too much for that.

Forever, my darling,

Your Da

18 August 1983

My dearest, dearest Suze,

This is one of those stolen moments again. I am writing in the barn-like lobby of the Sheraton waiting for some guy I should see might pass by.

I guess too often I just rely on hunches, or is it hoping against hope, for a sudden stroke of good luck to happen? Perhaps, the latter, because much of my life seems to have been directed, if not governed, by such unexpected happenings, which either bailed me out of a somewhat unsuccessful or awkward situation or which meant a new opportunity for business, promotion. Or, better yet, a new lease on life!

That's what happened when I met you on that night flight from Abidjan to Paris. It was 1970. Do you remember the exact date? Sometimes I wish I could relive it all over again with foresight – what would I have done? Would I have tried to lure you into staying in Paris?

So much has happened since then and, as you, I feel as if we finally reached our culmination point, the plateau where we want to be – *coûte que coûte* – whether it brings supreme joy or agonizing pain. We have made the choice: this is it, this is love, this is the ultimate love we have both searched for in our lives.

Now, when I swim my one kilometer, whenever I can (twenty times back and forth), thinking with each stroke: she loves me… she loves me… she loves me… Oh, what bliss to know that you love me, and more than that, to know that at last you do believe in my love for you, and that you accept it at its full depth and value. Now we truly know each other, and that is something no one can ever take away from us.

Your letter was magnificent. I so well understood and appreciated your expressions of half-dazed confusion, joy and fear and pain and frustration and ecstasy, all rolled into one big blob of unfathomable dimensions: no shape, no color, nothing distinct and it is there words fail to describe our feelings, which keep us tumbling over each other with ever greater speed, gathering momentum, leading us God knows where.

Oh, how I know that feeling because it overtakes me too, time and again.

No, darling, I shall never stop loving you. I shall never take that away from you. Whatever may happen in the future, whatever direction either one of us may go, I shall love you forever, Darling – my light, my love, source of every beautiful thought and inspiration. Dream of dreams, but you are not just a dream, a metaphysical phenomenon, a reality, instead of flesh and blood, housing a most noble, sweet, pure spirit. I am looking at the pictures I made of you, and caress you with my eyes, hold you in my arms tenderly, and ruffle your curls with my hand. Drinking the ambrosia of your smiling eyes, expressing rapture, emotion, and the gladness of life.

You're so alive, so very, very alive. Eager to live, eager to learn, mature and yet malleable, willing to take on anything which may further enrich your life. I can see now, that at last you have opened the doors of your heart and being, both for giving and receiving. Gates and barbed wire of cynicism and fear have been trashed, trampled and removed— the road is clear. Intuitively, you are avoiding the pitfalls now, while choosing just the right stepping stones toward your ultimate goals. I love California too, especially your setting.

Let's enjoy now, for now, and as long as we can and, if God wills, forever!

No, I am not blind to realism. I know we have to go on living our lives, tend to our duties, and continue to behave like good citizens, earning our bread, and taking care of everyday chores. All of that doesn't preclude that we may remain in this euphoric state of peace, love, and contentment.

We'll meet again, rather sooner than later. As you, I would just love to do the most ordinary things together with you: let's take that ferry across the bay someday; let's go to another concert in S.F., let's go for a hike in the woods, or beach-combing, or swimming or picnicking, or whatnot. Let's buy Belle Haven. You've enhanced its beauty, my love.

Above all, let's be together as long as we can and live, live, live!

I love you darling, oh so much – forever.

Da

A SEASON OF MISTS

New York
JFK airport
August 29, 1983

My sweetest, dearest darling,

This trip came up only a few days ago; on Friday morning I was not even sure whether they would let me go. I wanted to call you at home, but never had a chance. I had to do so many things at home, after having been away for so many weeks and now taking off again. It's only a short trip. Leaving for Amsterdam now and will be there until Thursday. Then two days for meetings in London and on Saturday, back to Washington again.

How I have missed you, darling. The days without any token of communication with you are growing longer and longer again. Will I ever get used to it, to live without you?

Yes, I wish you were here, and that we were travelling together to Holland now, so I could show you my favorite places, like the heather in Gooiland, where I spent my adolescent years, roaming around, spying on birds and deer and various small mammals. I collected plants for my herbarium – Wageningen on the Rhine – where I canoed and swam, and plodded through those endless pastures; then the lovely old towns of Delft, Leiden, Gouda, Alkmaar, but above all, my beloved Amsterdam. We'd see the sunset over the North Sea and bicycle through the dunes, and whiz by those pastures, looking at the constantly changing gray skies.

Suze, I love you, and may God give that someday, yes, someday, we can do just that, enjoy Holland as only a true Dutchman can.

I finally got the pictures back, which I took on my last trip. I had them done over again (they admitted at the photo shop that they had done a bum job). I am sending you only one of yourself (one I had made double) for now, that is. I have four others, which are even better. Oh, how I love them! Many, many a time during the day, I pull them out of my desk drawer, and sit there staring lovingly at your pictures, caressing your hair and smiling back into your radiant, joyous eyes. My secretary returned from vacation today, and I couldn't wait to show her the shots. I was so proud of them. She gasped, and said, "Oh, she is so *beautiful!*" I couldn't but agree wholeheartedly.

The other pictures of me are a bit of an experiment. I took them on the balcony of my hotel in Lima, Peru. They are my reflection in the semi-finish of the French door leading to the balcony. They are not very good, but you may still like them. It is just as well not to see me clearly but darkly and somewhat mysterious and vague, eh?

Darling, I love you and I must control myself, not to become too impatient when you don't write or call me. How about surprising me with a letter again, my love?

Would you like to take some time to come here to Washington between October 12 and 15?

Please write darling. I miss you and the desire to hold you in my arms burns like an everlasting flame. I am mad for you.

"There is the heat of Love, the pulsing rush of Longing, the lover's whisper, irresistible—magic to make the sanest man go mad."

Forever,
Da

A SEASON OF MISTS

Washington
September 9, 1983

My dearest love,

I called your home this morning (7:15 a.m. your time) and got a somewhat flustered teen on the line. Poor girl, I guess she was as embarrassed as I was and, yet I had the temerity to ask where you were. All she would say is that you wouldn't be back until Saturday.

A pity, I so much hoped to hear your voice again, soft, appealing with a tinkle of laughter in it. I miss you and I long for you. Loneliness is settling in again with that damned empty P.O. box staring me in the face each day, day after day, when I make my regular round at lunchtime. (I hope you did get my letter written on August 29 at JFK airport.)

Ever so many times I've looked at the few photos I have of you, caressing your face with my eyes, almost ready to lay my hand on your arm, be close to you just to let you know I am there.

Why do I want to continue to love you so much, while each thought, each flare-up of desire brings such unbearable pain in unison with something divinely blissful, which others may call happiness or gratification or contentedness. Ah, how bittersweet is my love. Yes, I will continue to love you all my life as you said you would do towards me. Better this than no love. Life would be too bloody tedious, dull, flat, and colorless without this love.

I guess it is the fulfilment of our life, this love; the fulfillment of all our hope, desires, plans and promises, of all the good and beautiful we have ever prayed for and dreamed about. Truth too (the old Roman/Christian goal of *verum bonum pulchrum*) especially after our last get together. I am more than ever struck by your intensity of honesty, goodness, devotion, truthfulness. I also keep rereading your last letter and don't know whether to cry or jubilate. It is so beautiful, your outpouring of love, confusion, devotion, yearning... ah, you and I... we're both caught, chained to each other and no one but no one can do anything about or against that. Just, you and I.

I don't know why I'm writing you all this. I don't want to confuse you. All I want to say over and over again that I love you my darling and that I miss you, and that being human and weak, I would like to hear from you now and then, some confirmation of your own feelings and just a little sign of life so I will know that you are all right, and happy and fully alive.

I know, I know you are busy and I am sure, you are still going through a very difficult time, considering the palavers of lawyers and family affairs that need straightening out.

Please forgive, therefore my impatience. It's just that I do love you so much that life without you is nothing more than a clock ticking away.

Darling, Darling, please write me, if only just a few words.

I miss you so much!

Da

"These letters, going back and forth about whether or not to stay tied to each other, they're actually the evidence of their commitment to each other. That's quite a price your mom paid. What was she, thirty-nine?"

"For me, his commitment to writing her makes him seem more authentic. He stays with her as she grows and matures, through all her misgivings, even when she tells him to go to hell. He doesn't believe her, but turns right around sending her that very letter back. It seems settled here, and there's less agonizing. Except that she doesn't write as often as he'd like."

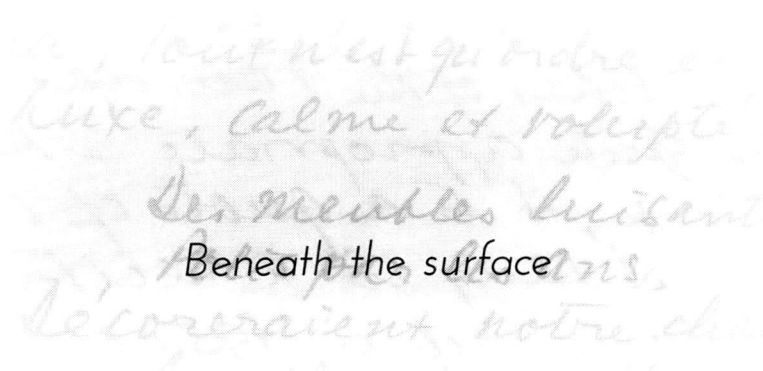

Beneath the surface

Wednesday
September 28, 1983

My dearest Suze,

You're probably right, I should not visit the post office daily. Somehow, my noontime walks inexplicably keep drawing me in that direction and once in the neighborhood, I cannot help but stop in the P.O. itself. I keep finding excuses: "Well, she did promise, didn't she?" "The mail is slow, a letter will come this week, if not today, it'll be there tomorrow"; "wonders never cease"; "fate will be kind to me this time," and so forth.

Ah well, so be it. You are just too caught up in your present hundreds of involvements.

Fall is on its way. It was pretty cold a week ago, but the past few days it's been sunny and clear and bright again; only the nights are growing colder and colder. It's Indian summer weather and just gorgeous. Wish you were here! You're *sure* you won't come between the eleventh and fourteenth of October?

I have no immediate plans for travel. The Thailand mission is still loosely scheduled for November; other than that, nothing's imminent for the time being. I still have to write umpteen reports on previous visits; I never seem to get through my backlog.

Thanks to this past summer and all the swimming I did, I feel nineteen years younger than when I first re-met you in May '81. (All those letters and no chance to see you.) Not only physically, but also mentally and you have played an important part in that rejuvenation process! Oh, Suze, I love you so much! Not because of that, but because you are you, a most magnificent creature, so lovely, so sweet, so endearing, so noble, so strong, so honest, so everything!

Yes, I love you, Darling and I wish you were here! All my love and tenderness...

Forever, Your Da

Oct. 4, 1983
En route Amsterdam – Istanbul

My dearest Suze,

The mini-vacation is over again, and I'm on my way to Turkey. I will write you a long letter as soon as I can, but right now I just want to drop you a few lines that, in spite of having spent a rather idyllic and pleasant vacation, which included a tour of southern England, your image has followed me wherever I have gone. I have thought of you daily/hourly, compared notes and often wished I could do it all over again with you at my side!

I love you deeply, Suze and keep hoping against all reality that someday you and I will be together permanently, inseparable, belonging to each other, enjoying all things together. I love you, and I cannot help myself. I love you and will continue to love you forever. Is it me or another me? I don't know. All I know is that you are a part of me already, if not physically, at least spiritually. You occupy far too much time/space/volume of my inner emotional life to be considered a mere friend or occasional lover . I consider you "mine", and hence, have no fear, don't doubt for a moment that I will not try everything in my power to get together with you, as soon and as often as I can.

Yours forever, Da

Potomac, Maryland
Friday, October 15, 1983

My love, my one and only,

It was storming last night and now at 9:00 a.m. the sun is shining, the world seems to be at peace, the maples turning red, a fall nip in the air… it's just beautiful! So beautiful that one could wish to share it with another – you and I – but I am alone and so are you. And we both yearn and long for each other.

Lover, it is not the thought and desire of making love to you that keeps me going. True, it is a very important part of it, insofar as it is the culmination of everything at the end of being together for a while, at the end of holding hands, looking into each other's eyes, absorbing all the beauty within and without us, of listening to music, man-made and nature-made. How I love to hear: raindrops (you, I'm sure, remember) playing their staccato tune on a tin roof, the wind whistling through pine trees, the steady splash of a creek with little falls; the song of a lark; or the sad, nostalgic coo of a mourning dove. Yes, at the end of a day filled with impressions like that, during which we grow closer and closer together and the longing becomes more acute, and the desire to become one becomes almost unbearable, yes, I would like to take you in my arms and fondle and caress you, cover you with kisses, cover you with my body and melt into unison with you. Let my heart pound next to your heart, my breath mingle with yours, my tears flow with your tears, our gasps unite into a song of love, of total self-sacrifice in the name of love and adoration. Oh, how I love you. My loins ache for this, the ultimate expression of the gift of one's self.

I must say in spite of the wonderful conversation we had last night, I slept rather restlessly. You were with me all night long. I could almost feel the touch of your hand. I kept hearing your voice over and over again, "I love you, I love you, Da."

Will you ever believe me truly and unshakably that I love you as much as I do? Believe me it isn't easy. Now that you are free, I want to love you (and I do), but at times it hurts as much as it delights. No, love, you are not the only one suffering by it.

But I gladly suffer for this, knowing we have a love like this. But, my God, what did you do to me to make me love you that much? Sometimes, my angel, it is almost unbearable. We must go on living our lives... alas, our separate lives.

Your Da

On board an Alitalia jet
October 25, 1983

My dearest, sweetest love,

Guess what? I am en route to Abidjan, sitting next to a young (Dutch) mother of two little girls. She's on her way to Kano, where her husband is the Alitalia representative – a bit reminiscent of the memorable trip to Paris, from Abidjan, in February 1970! Except that:

You, in spite of your illness looked young and fresh and optimistic and desirable and this woman looks haggard and worn out, even though she's probably no older than thirty.

You are you and she is she and there's no comparison, because you are and will ever be the most beautiful and appealing and sweet and desirable woman in my life, now and forever.

Non, l'histoire ne ce repète pas…

It would be different, if you were here again next to me, thirty or forty thousand feet above the earth, loose from daily chores and worries, high up in the air, close to the angels and God. You and me, finally finding your hand when the baby slept, stroking your back and we talked all the night. Oh how I wish I could do it all over again, except that I wouldn't stop in Paris anymore. I'd go on with you to Geneva, Lausanne, wherever… the end of the world, if you would wish just to be with you to love you and take care of you forever.

Kairos pei, panta rei . Real life keeps flowing, and we are carried in life's stream which keeps carrying us on and on, forever on and on down, as all streams do. Occasionally we hit a pool, a widening in the stream, and for a moment, or while, the stream loses its impetus, milling us around, slowly, undecidedly, giving us time to breathe a little, to think, to take stock and to gather strength for the next journey, down and down, and forever on and on. No, we cannot look back; it's behind us. We've passed that ridge, that crest; it has joined the land of dreams and memories now. It's reality we are facing again, the sharp rocks underneath the water's surface, which hurt us when we bump against them; the overhanging branches of trees whipping our faces and bodies, like the seemingly impenetrable intertwined and twisted roots of the mangrove trees in our way, causing us to close our eyes temporarily and abandon ourselves to the mercy of nature's force and God's goodwill.

On and on, we flow trying to shape our destiny against all odds and being successful only part of the time, because sheer willpower makes us jump the hurdles and divert our course in the maelstrom. On and on we go, hoping that it all will end well, that we will reach that placid, peaceful pool at the end surrounded by palms and orchids and tranquility. Peace, calm beauty, rest – the final pool, where no alligators or water snakes lurk on their prey, where colorful fish and coral complete the scene of serenity, where we *know* that the end of the journey, this haven, this fulfilled promise made it all worthwhile.

I guess what I mean to say is there's a lot outside of us that moves us, drives us, determines our lives for us, and there's not much we can do about that. But, Suze there's also us, our inner selves, our determination and will, which helps us to overcome some of the hurdles, which gives us a fighting chance to direct our own destiny and life's setting… the inevitable stream. We must *not* give up because we have that chance, and we must be on our *qui vive* to utilize that chance at all times,

Why am I so philosophical? I guess it's the altitude, the setting. For a moment I had to redirect my gaze at this woman next to me. Alas, no, it is not you. Oh Suze, how can I ever stop loving you, centering my daily life now and in the future on you? I really don't want to stop because I love you. I love you so very much, that you are my life and life without you becomes unbearable.

I am closing my eyes to the future insofar as it involves you, because, to be realistic, it is obvious I will have to lose you someday; that I have to let you go out of my life. The image of you, sweet, lovely you, will gradually loosen itself from my mind, dissolve in the mist, overhanging that stream of our life, your face will melt into splashes of light and dark leaving me alone to carry on forever by myself. Then, then will it be worth the struggle to fight on, to direct and redirect, to avoid the obstacles in my path, or shall I wash up on a shore, lost to life?

You are the grand obsession of my life, *la grande illusion*, the magnificent sorcerer of my dreams and desires, the gist and color of my life. Without you, everything would be gray and tasteless, dull and boring. No, I won't think of it, not yet. Oh, God, let a miracle happen. Let it all change, let her become mine *forever*. Hear my prayer, let her be mine, mine, mine! No, I cannot live without you . You drive me, inspire me, arouse me, fill me with thoughts, dreams, desires... you are my muse. You are my life's focal point, the very center, the core of my being and *raison d'etre*. No, I am not exaggerating. No one can tell me my mind, my thinking, my ego – only I can do so and, I swear that's the way I feel and think.

Oh, love, my dear sweet Suze. You are so, oh so, desirable, so loveable, so huggable. Perhaps no one ever told you so but I do. I, whose mind and spirit has captured you. I, who am possessed by you and your image.

Even though you are alone now, and he is in the past, I beg you, don't give up on me... not yet. Not too soon. Maybe a miracle will happen. Maybe it will all come true. Maybe you will be mine, and we'll be together.

Am I no longer in the realm of reason? It is not that I am dreaming. I am wishing. As a boy, I firmly believed that if one wanted something strongly enough, one would get it. Mind over matter.

Perhaps, perhaps I will be granted that one fervent wish, the wish of a lifetime, the ultimate wish. I don't even want to think what the result will be. It will be total bliss and ecstasy, rapture, the sublimation of all human desires.

I am running out of superlatives. I must stop. I am boring you, no doubt. You have heard it all before, from me, at least!

In conclusion, you know what I mean, at least I'm trusting that you do. I do love you more, more than a mere mortal can express. You are the embodiment of paradise, of the ultimate peace, desire, and fulfillment. You are you, after all these years, and you are the fantastic, the beautiful, the truth, the perfect good and virtue to me.

I love you, I love you, I love you and I'll never stop loving you. In the brightness of day and the darkness of night, in the glow of success, and the depression of failure, in the shining future and with *aussichtslos* (hopeless) present, you are the beacon, the steady light, the solid immovable rock on which I will always be able to trust and build.

I love you... forever.

Your Da

P.S. Tomorrow I will be fifty-nine.

High water

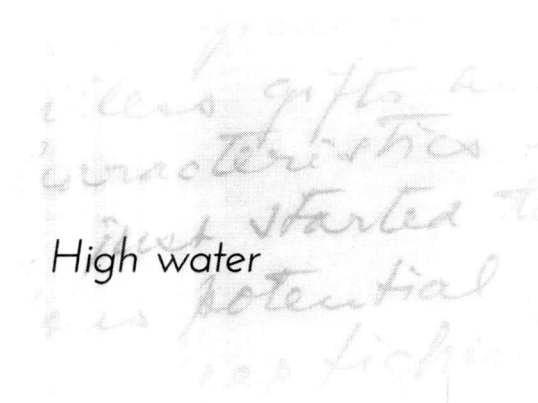

3 November 1983
My dearest Love,

No, even though the stationery comes from the Hyatt in San Francisco, I'm no longer in S.F. but Paris. Here I am, sitting by myself in one of those highly touted restaurants, Le Pied de Cochon, (I am not disappointed). I am all by myself, holding long conversations with you sitting across the table from me, holding your hand, and trying to touch your knee.

I wish it were 1970, instead of 1983. Perhaps that is not true either, because even in 1971, and even though I was all aflame for you, I did not realize yet what a wonderful gem you were. Will you ever forgive me?

Time and again, this week, I have been thinking about you, as always, but, particularly in the context of the letter I wrote you on the Alitalia plane.

Often we, or rather, I, will confuse happenings in past time with the reality of the present, or more precisely, with what the thoughts and feelings were at that particular time compared to the present. I know this thought isn't clear, but I'll go on.

That night in the plane, I was indeed *bouleversé* (turned upside down) by you. I was so crazy about you I could have eaten you, so to say. Yet, by the end of that trip, when we said good-bye in that early foggy morning at Paris, I was convinced that that was the end. Not that I wished it to end, on the contrary, but it was so unexpected and beautiful, like a dream. I thought of us as, pardon the cliché, ships passing in the night. I couldn't dare to think we would ever see each other again.

When I kissed you good-bye, you were reluctant, and then with such great tenderness, you responded to me. I handed over your baby, and she put her face in your neck as I would have liked to have done. She was asleep there against you when you walked away with your son and a heap of stuff to manage.

You gave me your address in Geneva where you would be staying briefly with your sister-in-law to see a Swiss doctor who could treat your kidney infection. (For sure, Abidjan was no place to be treated.) But I had no address or information for you after you reached California where you would be furloughing, completely well by then, I hoped, and reunited with David. Then I opened the little red backpack I had forgotten to give you, while kissing you and all and there was the address, your actual physical address!

Obviously, you received my letter in Geneva, and, in no time at all, I was holding a response from you, a perfect reflection of my own awe and wonder at our meeting and that conversation through the night.

Next came the meeting on Mount Diablo. You were reluctant to embrace an affair unless it could come to fruition. How stupid of me not to realize that, me, still in my highly scrupulous stage (we Catholics are all alike with our guilt syndrome), and not wanting to make implausible promises, which might implode on contact, promises I could not keep. We said good-bye again.

A SEASON OF MISTS

Moving to Kenya, I could not get you out of my mind. I did everything I could to contact you when I came to the States during two successive annual leaves. At last, upon my return to Washington, we were able to be in touch again, even though by then you were back in Africa. I finally found you through your church, and was devastated that you were gone again.

Again, two years ago, (two and a half by now) I almost began to feel the same as I did in 1971, as if I should hope. You were hesitant, knowing in your mind what you wanted and needed, but not yet courageous enough to act on it, that is, a divorce.

In the meantime, I grew fonder and fonder of you. I really got you under my skin and that's where you are now, and, in spite of the hopelessness of the situation, I began to love you so much. Now, I cannot stop myself anymore!

Finally your decision to divorce, which first came as an ominous blow to me and then almost simultaneously opened up new vistas: you would be free soon, and it would be up to me to make you mine.

In the meantime, I let my feeling and dreams and wishes go full speed, pulling out all the stops, so to speak. And I have become a victim of my own lack of control. Now where am I? I love you so much, it tears me apart. Instead of keeping me in a constant state of exhilaration, it can pull me down. I don't want to see you alone or with anyone else but myself.

I thought then that you would be free soon. It would be up to me to make you mine. But conscience plays its part again. What do I have to offer, really? I am getting long in the tooth as they say.

The fact remains that *you* were the instigator of your new life. You wanted to be free, not in my cage, but free as a bird.

You made that very clear to me. "Let go, and stay out of my life, Da," you said. Instead, I kept hounding you, begging you, loving you more and more. My God, how I want you for my own. I have never felt more possessive in my life.

Instead of giving you continuing support and love, I keep on hurting you.

Forever, Da

November 14, 1983

My Darling,

And so I wrote in Paris. I was so desperate and felt miserable, with a bad cold, bronchitis, asthma and fever. I felt lonelier than ever. Yes, desperate is the word. For somehow I felt I had to make a decision, there and then and that there was only one way out: to stop it all!

Now, I am not so sure. I must say when I received your letter written following David's visit I felt like crying with you. I was greatly moved, having been reminded again how great the turmoil must be for you at present. Sometimes I feel so very guilty for trying to persuade you to keep on loving me. You have enough on your hands to bother with that too. But then I talk myself into believing that I just may be a source of consolation and inspiration for you and bestow some love on you, put salve on the wound.

Do I?

Whatever, I love you and I want your happiness so tell me and when I am in the way, making it impossible for you to achieve that happiness. Please tell me!

A SEASON OF MISTS

Now that you are free, should I become a bigamist, a Mormon? Shall I live two separate lives? Frankly, those are not workable solutions either.

I love you come hell or high water. I love you and will keep on loving you, even if it tears me apart. I will do everything for you to make you happy except divorce "C." She has all those held-over fears of the war years.

You can count on my love forever and ever. Do with it what you like. If you want to have me out of your life and soul forever, say so. And I shall hold my tongue from here on, forever too!

I want you to know three basic things:

    a. I love you
    b. I know you love me, and
    c. I only want your happiness, not my own.

My love is yours my dearest, sweetest darling, my nymph, my real dream (a long waited for reality, I mean). My inspiration, my muse, my lovely…

Forever, Your Da

On the beach

December 20, 1983

My Darling Suze,

If I don't write right now (7:30 a.m. at the office), I won't get around to it until Christmas I'm afraid. So, here it goes in the hope it will reach you in time.

Unfortunately, there won't be much time to write you a long letter, for I have a board presentation (of the Rwanda tea project) today, and I still have to prepare myself for that one. Besides, I am trying to get at least a draft of my appraisal report on the banana, limes, pineapple project in the Ivory Coast finished before Christmas. I had hoped to utilize this month of December to get through my backlog of the calendar year. Instead, the backlog has been growing while I sit here behind my desk. And, for next year (1984) there is a horrendous work and travel program: Mexico, Paraguay (at least three projects) Brazil, maybe Argentina, Ivory Coast, Cameroon (two projects), Kenya, Mali, Rwanda, Zambia, Tanzania (maybe), Uganda, Sudan, Turkey, Thailand (two projects), Dominican Republic, and undoubtedly a few others which will pop up at the last moment.

Enough about work. I am planning visits with you as I go.

A SEASON OF MISTS

How are you, my Darling? I hope you will receive your Christmas package before the big day. Since you are free now, it brings me joy to send you small gifts. I'll always keep you in the perfume I gave you at our first meeting at Mt. Diablo, that is: *Je Reviens* (I will return) by Worth. I so much hope that your Christmas will be serene and peaceful, and the upcoming New Year will be the greatest ever for you. I am proud of you, the way you have taken charge of your own life.

I could go on raving about you. No wonder since we were together I lie awake at nights, thinking of you, desiring you, lusting for you. No wonder I keep dreaming the impossible dream, to have and to hold you forever and ever, to cherish you, protect you, take care of you, love you, hug you in an everlasting embrace, enjoy life with you: nature, art, music, sounds, leaves of grass, flowers, birds, sunshine and rain, waves, wind, heather, forest, alps and fjords, the corners of the world, crowds and solitude, everything and all things… You are the pivot of my thinking, my dreams, my desires, my life.

No matter what happens, no matter how long we will be kept separated through circumstances and all factors within and beyond our control, I shall always love you, Suze, my dearest, sweetest, loveliest Suze.

Again, my heart cries out for you.

I love you, Darling,

Hugs and kisses

Yours forever, Da

January 22, 1984

My dearest love, the muses have not inspired me to write you a long and loving letter. As a matter of fact, I feel numb and slightly mad. Let me hasten to say not with you. Oh, no, far from that. No, it's because of the stupidity of the airlines, which put exact arrival and departure times in the schedules, down to the last minute and yet, you're lucky if you make it one hour (in the summer) or two or three hours (in winter).

I arrived at Dulles airport in good time this afternoon to catch the 2:45 to New York. However, I was told the first flight had been cancelled. Instead, they squeezed me into an overfilled and rickety bus, which took me clear over to National Airport to take a 3:45 flight. Well, we got there and were told our flight to Paris would leave within one hour. After two gate changes, we've been told our flight won't leave earlier than 8:30. Oh, the charm and excitement of travel.

Anyway, there's a good chance my baggage may be with me on the same plane. But, let's hope I'll make the connection to Abidjan.

I promised you I would fill you in on my exploits. Well, I haven't been in very good shape since about December 20. I got the same excruciating pains in my side and lower abdomen again, the same as those I had when I picked up a good amoebic dysentery in Turkey at the end of '82. I have spent two days at the doctor's office in some radiology, x-ray or ultrasound lab. All tests were negative, everything is fine, but I couldn't sleep because of the constant jabbing pain, which felt like my insides were being torn out. In the meantime I had all sorts of visions, of having cancer of the liver or the colon. Actually, once I tuned myself in to the real possibility, I was surprised how relatively easy and willing I was to accept it!

A SEASON OF MISTS

Amazingly, two days ago, the pain suddenly disappeared, and I feel relatively fit again and ready to travel.

In a way though, an interesting experience, because once more I was able to face death squarely and openly and in the final analysis I gained a much greater appreciation of life and life's beauty. Images of you moved through my mind, especially your smile.

Even with the cold, icy weather here, I enjoyed walking the dog every evening, at sunset and again close to midnight with a full moon hanging in the sky and shedding its bright light on the snow. One early evening, I stood in wonder, looking out over the area where we live, from the top of a hill, facing our house on the corner and suddenly I saw the whole scene as one large magnificent Currier and Ives painting. I was transported, and thought myself living a century earlier. When I tore myself away from that picture, I realized I had created another image of nostalgia in my memory file; many are connected to you. Coming back and forth from work I have been playing (by tape) Rachmaninoff's music exclusively for about two weeks now. It somehow fitted my mood and ushered me forward to think of us.

I'll be looking forward to receive a letter from you in Paris. Please, don't let me wait in vain, Suze my love.

I'll write you again in more mellow a mood.

I love you. You know that. Don't forget. I also hope you are well, my sweetheart, and that this year, indeed, will begin to bring you the fulfillment of your fondest wishes and dreams.

Love, love and love again,

Forever, Your Da

P.S. In case you lost it: Scribe Hotel, 1, Rue Scribe, 75009 Paris France

Telex 214653, Tel. 742-0304

January 23, 1984

My Darling Da,

You'll have arrived in Paris by now, the first leg of another long journey. Your journeys always seem a little sad to me, almost as if you set out to experience a deeper loneliness, but perhaps to know yourself better and experience that heightened sense of selfhood. You're very much in touch with your feelings, and conscious of your love for me in a way I find reassuring and touching.

I always ache for you a little more or differently while you're away, wondering if you're well, hoping you're not drowning any of your sorrows or overexerting. (You're in marvelous condition, by the way.) I work at it more faithfully than I did; it's more play than work because I'm inspired by the ocean and the brisk weather of the season here in Santa Cruz.

You are away and in touch with a greater, bigger world. I can visualize you, your neatly packed bags, everything compartmentalized. Sometimes, I'm frightened by your fastidiousness.

And me, I'm here longing for you, the feelings get all bunched up with the crazy fears that seize me in the evenings. Now is when the longing gives space to the reality, when the sun sets and I come inside. You run with me on the beach, or did you know? Were you here, I should like to be held for hours, yet how can I even know that you would read my mood. Just how would we experience life together with me, so unformed, an ugly fledgling. I'm like a blob of clay, too dried out to shape. God, for all the times I spent in churches, five meetings a week for how many years? I utter prayers, but leave my totally worn Bible orphaned on the shelf.

I wonder sometimes how Milton felt, blind and in despair at the end. Paradise lost. I have been reading *Passages* by Gail Sheehy. Have you heard of this book? I've been down many paths, me the runaway, the mid-life-crisis casualty.

Thank God for routine: milk cartons go dry, the wash accumulates, kids need to do homework and be fed. So you call and take me to Paris for a moment in my imagination. I close out everything except your voice.

You're there in another time zone, and I wish your nights corresponded to mine, that you turned while alone to think of me. How delicately you touched me. I've never been loved so intimately. I want you so much this evening, my love, my lifelong love.

Suze

March 20, 1984

Suze,

The first day of spring and my heart skips a beat when I look at the crocuses popping out of my little grass-patch near the fish pond, when I smell resin in the air, when I see the Forsythia branches leaf out, when I feel the sun softly glowing on my face… Promises of more to come. Promises, promises.

Yes, the euphoria would be complete if only you were at my side but you are so far, and so am I.

I love you Suze and miss you oh so badly.

Your Da

May 2, 1984

My faraway dream girl,

Paris again, misty, watery, gray and melancholic. It must have been that way about fourteen years ago when I left you at Orly, when I had to say adieu. Your face is still haunting me when I make my endless walks through these boulevards and little, narrow side streets; and I keep hoping against all hope, as unrealistic as it is, that I will see you.

Someday, yes, someday we'll have a chance to do it all over again, together this time. Oh, Paris again would be bliss with you. Instead, I am in the most melancholic frame of mind.

Love, oh so much love,

Da

P.S.: Letter is following soon!

The ark

"The Ark"
Aberdare Mountains
Kenya
Sunday night

Suze, my all,

I say "my all" because you embody everything that is dear to me: love, unison, inspiration, hope, desire, beauty, femininity but above all the ideal woman... *mi mujer*. I dreamed last night of you. It was a sad dream and I was very confused. I was running back and forth from home to some unknown place, a very public place, full of people, although I didn't notice all these people because I was searching for you, saw you, lost you again, finally I sat down with you and another person. You were talking while I was trying to make eye contact with you. Lots of things were happening – people coming and going, including yourself.

Finally, you returned and announced to me that you were leaving with this stranger. You looked sad, and we kissed. We embraced very fondly while everyone was looking on then I fled, I ran away, without looking back, while somebody else was trying to keep up with me, looking sideways at me and I kept going faster and faster because I was embarrassed, because I was crying, tears running down my cheeks. And the more people looked at me, the more I cried because I realized this was the end, the end of any meaningful life because I had lost you… lost you forever.

I woke up crying and kept thinking of that dream all day.

I thought of you all day, as I do every day. You are at my side, and with each thing I do, or experience I try to imagine how you would react.

I always proclaim that I will not change my life for anything, that I'd rather have the ups and downs associated with loving you, than having no love at all and yet, at times I wonder whether the heartache associated with not being able to call you my own and the fear of losing you eventually will not be my final undoing. The hurt, my love, is sometimes getting the better of me, so often I feel like crying out in the idle hope that you would hear me and run to my side. The pain in my chest becomes unbearable. Yes, it is almost physical, that pain. I'm serious – once you reach sixty, and once you have been face to face with death, the fear of dying stays with you no matter how well you may feel at a particular moment.

I was reading an article on pain in *TIME*, and realized that pain as such is no longer an issue with me. I can stand pain very well. I have experienced it in many forms and manifestations. For me, the problem with pain is only that it is associated with dying and/or death and although I felt strangely at ease with the thought of dying last winter, and was ready to accept the fact that I was, after all, not immortal, I am now back to my old stand: that I still have many, many years to live, the main reason being that I want to have a chance to live a "second" life, in which you Suze, will be my *one and only!*

But again, pain is not my problem. It is the asthma now. Asthma does not hurt, not at all, but the mere fact that you cannot breathe does send you in a panic, and often makes you believe that death is imminent.

I now wake up in the middle of the night, almost nightly between 2:00 or 3:00 a.m., gasping for breath. Often, I am not even able to inhale the medicine from the vaporizer I keep at my side because my whole breathing ability seems to have come to a halt. After several tries, I succeed, but it may take an hour or more before I can breathe more or less normally again, and lie down to sleep. Whether or not I eventually will fall asleep is another matter…

Somehow, American doctors seem to think that one or two specific drugs, or a combination of several, are all that's needed to keep asthma under control. In a way, they are right. I can keep it more or less under control; but I want more: I want a cure. After having suffered at least thirty years, off and on, from asthma, I am convinced that one should be able to cure whatever it is that triggers asthma attacks in a person. Each person, admittedly, reacts differently, and the trigger mechanism is not only different from person to person, but may change over the years for the same person. As most physicians take the easy way out, they just prescribe some medicines and let it go at that. That's why I believe an institute devoted exclusively to lung disease and disorders will do more than that. That's why I would like to submit myself to the intensive care at the National Asthma Center to get over this damnable disease, once and for all!

After almost a week of touring all over Kenya, we finally ended up tonight at "The Ark", a famous lodge in the Aberdare Mountains National Park where the guests can watch wildlife day and night from glassed in verandas and bunkers. It is 1:00 a.m. now, and I got myself strategically located in the corner of the veranda where I have just enough light to write (a reflection of the spotlights trained on the salt-licks area), while also being able to watch the game. Since I sat here, practically alone (except for one couple and a Japanese fellow who is trying to learn English from the Kenyan barkeeper), for the last two hours or so, there's been a constant procession of animals: a huge bull elephant, two hyenas, a civet cat, a buffalo, two bush bucks, a hare. It's fascinating! They all come to lick the salt and take their time. The elephant is obviously the master – whenever the buffalo shows up, he chases him away – the hyenas and bush bucks come and go, but stay a respectful distance from him.

Again, I hear myself talk to you, and hear you whispering in my ear, while your lovely head rests on my shoulder. Methinks, there's so much we would enjoy together!

Since we left Kenya five years ago, the same hotel chains that manage this lodge (and several similar ones) apparently set up a very fancy, highly secluded private club (accommodations for twenty-four persons only) at the coast. I have decided that that's the place where I shall abduct you someday.

Are you game?

I just sat by the fireplace for a while to warm up. It's winter now in Kenya, and at seven thousand feet, it gets mighty cool at night. The animals have gone. The hoped for Rhino did not show up, after all. We saw a glimpse of him earlier in the evening but the people were making too much noise at that time. It's past 2:00 a.m. now, and I guess I had better hit the sack, like the pack of white-tailed mongoose that showed up a while ago, side by side, cozily keeping each other warm.

I wish you were here, so we could bed down side by side in the still of the night, broken only by the cry of a bird, the bark of a hyena, and the satisfied grunting of the elephant. They provide a hot water bottle here.

I love you so much, it hurts. I miss you so much, and that hurts even more. I wish you were here, and sometimes, in my wildest dreams you are suddenly there or here, rather with me, holding my arms, touching my cheeks with your lips, oh so gently, as you have, just being there being you… *mi mujer.*

Nairobi
21 June (Thursday)

We returned Monday night to the city, have been in meetings ever since, with the sponsors of the project we are appraising (Unilever) and the other interested co-financiers ad nauseam, except for yesterday when I flew with three others to a town near the Kenya/Uganda border in a chartered plane. Quite an adventure, for upon arrival, or near arrival it appeared that the landing gear of the Piper Seneca plane did not work. We had some anxious fifteen minutes, circling over the air strip, until the pilot reasoned that the wheels were out, but that the relay switches turning on the red danger light were at fault. Thank God he was right, but in the meantime, I could only think of you and that we would never live together.

On the way back to Nairobi, we got into one hell of a squall and tropical rainstorm. The plane bounced around so much, we were afraid it was going to break apart. Well, we made it, but I swore I was never going to fly one of those petite affairs anywhere, ever!

I am wrapping up my business here tomorrow. The others are staying on, but I feel I have sized it up sufficiently, and there's no need to gather any more data. There are always eager beavers who want to keep on collecting figures!

So, I'd better mail this tomorrow from here, because I'll be stopping in Italy (Sardinia) for four days, and the postal service in that country is even less reliable than the one here.

I am looking forward to some rest. I am dead tired, worn out. I haven't slept more than three to four hours per night since I came here, because of the pressure of work and the nightly bout of asthma.

Suze, oh how I wish you were here. Just being with you would uplift my spirits to such an extent, that nothing would bother me at all, nothing at all. I can just imagine me sitting here scanning once more the data we gathered here, while preparing myself for a final "exposé" tomorrow, in an attempt to persuade the sponsors and my colleagues to radically restructure the project – it is unworkable the way they have presented it to us – while you are already lying in bed, reading or dozing, listening to the (taped) classical music of the hotel room radio or sitting up in bed. You'd be facing me (sitting in an easy chair surrounded by stacks of paper), looking at me with your lovely eyes, and me caressing (with my eyes) your breasts and nipples shining through your nightie...

At last, I would put the papers away and join you in bed, holding you in my arms, feeling your soft skin against mine, your hair tickling my face, whispering endearments to each other, realizing and savoring the goodness of life together.

Will we ever?

I would like to keep on writing, but I must stop; it is midnight, and I have another heavy day coming up tomorrow, before boarding the night flight to Rome twenty-four hours from now. Oh, the romance of travel and adventure... hmmm!

I love you, Suze, go to sleep, my darling. I'll kiss your eyes, sweet dreams. Come nestle yourself in my arms, rest peacefully and know that you are safe with me because...

I love you,

Da

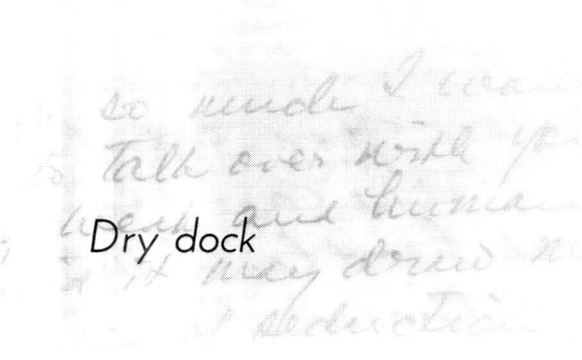

Dry dock

1 October 1984
En route Salt Lake City – Washington

My Lover...

Just reread (over and over again) your last few letters, including the "Mahlerian" one (as I'd like to call it), crying out as only you can in response to my baring my thoughts in a letter written in solitude in a simple hotel room in Buenos Aires.

You express the same feelings I have experienced for so long in a constant wondering about their ironic occurrence: The feelings of pain, of desertion, of such intensity that it reduces our whole being to a feared and yet willing submission to martyrdom. Why do we willingly accept this torture, which is the direct creation and result of our overwhelming love and desire for each other? Why does it have to hurt so much to love? Why do we, in the end, even find delight in the stabbing and tearing apart of our inner soul and heart?

We are truly romantics and can therefore unify our thoughts with Rachmaninoff, Mahler, Monet, Rodin, Goethe and those who went before us; trying to put in music, in paintings, words, poems the same emotions and heart-quakes, we, the more sensitive souls of the world continue to experience and wonder about! When you paint, you go all inside yourself, and the prize is a wonderful creation I could not have imagined. I do see your pain in them sometimes, like the great master El Greco, the dark colors, the elongated bodies and faces.

As far as I know, there's nothing we can do about it other than making the (unwanted) decision of trying to forget each other, to stop loving each other. But how can we? Apart from the fact that I find it impossible to forget you, I am willing to pay the price and sacrifice concomitant with the gift (giving and receiving) of love.

As you know, my mission to the Dominican Republic was canceled, because the sponsoring company (Castles and Cooke) was getting worried that we would become too deeply involved in their internal affairs while appraising a large cantaloupe project. It's their loss, as far as I can see, and it's no skin off my back (a strange phrase), although I was furious about the last minute cancelation after I had made all sorts of arrangements, including those for our getting together.

I now keep hoping and praying that the new plan will go through without a hitch. I have to be a few days in Fort Collins, Colorado, and Paul and I do have an investors' meeting planned near Denver, near the site of our new 3,000 head dairy farm, on October 20 and 21. I should be home on my sixtieth birthday (I have a hunch they are planning a surprise party for me) so the most likely days to plan a two-day trip to Davis, California would be either before or after October 20-21, and before the 26th. The Fort Collins and Denver stays should be in sequence too so the dates for a visit would have to be the 22nd and 23rd or 18th and 19th. I see now I have to attend a computer course in Washington on the 25th and 26th. I believe the 22–23 period is the best, so let's keep it that way! In that case, I could arrive on Sunday night, the 21st (Your 40th) and leave on the morning of the 24th. Let me know whether this is okay with you!

And then there is still the Las Vegas trip. We could either be together through that week, or a few days in the tail end – in other words November 25–30 or on the 29th and 30th in Las Vegas or I could come to Belle Haven. Please don't postpone the October chance until then. We should grab what we can at any and all times.

I was heartbroken myself for not being able to see you today. I do have a present, safely tucked in the bottom of my briefcase. Now, it will have to wait. Not for long, I hope.

It is hard to describe to you, and make you believe how much I become absorbed in planning such trips, where I hope to have a chance to meet you. Really, I lie awake trying to figure out the tiniest details. I scheme and scheme, coming up with grandiose scenarios, and trying to invent all sorts of alternatives until, bang, somebody throws a monkey wrench in the works and shatters all my plans and dreams.

Good God, don't let it happen again. Give us a break and let us become united in our love in the most perfect, balanced, deep and fully altruistic love, mankind has ever known!

I love you, my darling, more than I will ever be able to say in words. But, perhaps I can at least hint at, by my actions, when we are together!

Forever,

Your Da

"I don't remember a letter from Buenos Aires. But then, my God, unlike most men, he's always baring his soul," Ellie says.

"Your mom, El, seems to believe they were destined to be together. I'm so glad she has Belle Haven. Her studio has so much pure light; she can go there and be with him in her mind. Yesterday when she painted, her strokes were looser, less controlled. She may go a whole new direction. That can happen to people after a traumatic experience."

"I was surprised she painted so soon after his death. The colors are so muted. It tells on her that she may lose Belle Haven."

"Ellie, there's something I've noticed throughout. He never talks of his children with your mother. She rarely speaks of you two. As a psychologist, that seems significant to me. The world goes away for them in their fantasy of being together. He seems more obsessed than she, but still..."

> My dearest, dearest Suze
>
> I keep postponing writing to you. Why? Because rereading your letters, over and over, I realize the enormity of love and sacrifice and devotion you have poured into writing them, an effort of that deserves nothing but the very best (from my side), while at this point I cannot do much more than jot down a few thoughts because of the usual time constraints at the office, plus all the interruptions. (I started this exactly one hour ago, and a non-stop-stream of visitors, investment officers, et al., has kept me from making any progress whatsoever.) This afternoon, however, I decided that I at least should write you a few lines to let you know that I am thinking of you, and to assure you of my undying love. If anything, I love you more than ever, although each time I say this, I cannot believe that I could ever surpass the magnitude, depth, and intensity of my love for you.
>
> Strangely enough, after we said good-bye two weeks ago, I felt a great emptiness within and outside of me as if I had been cast out of a spaceship, into the great universe. For a very brief while, a few days later, I even noticed within myself a hesitatingly mute acceptance of the fact that I would have to live a life of barren loneliness from here on. I repressed all feeling of passion and desire, and whenever I thought of you (i.e. continuously) I forced myself to think of you a long-ago sweet memory, as if I met you in a spring-flowered pasture in one of my earlier years of existence as a butterfly alighting on

a flower, slowly waving its colorful, radiant wings, as if beckoning me to come near. A few days ago, the blood began to rush through my veins with renewed vigor (when I decided that sixty wasn't all that old, after all), and with it your image came back in force, haunting me, begging me, caressing me, arousing me, sending me in sweet oblivion and abandon. I think of myself in your arms, my head resting on your belly, my stroking, and caressing your soft skin, and lovely, curved backside (you have the most fascinating, adorable buttocks, my sweet!)

Yes, I lust for you as never before. I am getting sexually aroused each time I think of you. I swear, it is more often than I can bear but please don't think for a moment that my love has become merely, and entirely physical. The thoughts and desires described above are a mere expression of my overwhelming desire to be with you, as intimately as possible, so we may reunite in the most intimate way by baring our souls to each other, after having bared our bodies in each other's presence. We've always been able to talk easily together, from the start.

Before I close (I must run now, but shall write you again soon), just one more thing: you still underestimate my capability of understanding and commiserating. When you proposed to me I never thought for one moment, nor did it ever enter my mind, before or after our beautiful get together (on the 19th) that you would even think of financial or physical security, when asking me or accepting my love. I know you love me for what and who I am (as I do you), and I am exceedingly honored by that. Anything outside that is a mere *bagatelle*, which may or may not be important at those rare times, when there is a real need for it.

As I said, your letter deserves a much more grandiose treatment than I can give now but I didn't want to wBWait another day without letting you hear from me.

I am grateful to you, I adore you, I worship you. Yes, you are my life and I do accept your offer. I love you, my Darling. No, I do not want to say good-bye either. I love you too much for that.

Forever, your Da

And lover…

P.S. Yes, come to Las Vegas if you can, and for as long as you can. I will be there from Sunday November 25 (evening) until Friday, 30th.

Washington D.C.
November 19, 1984

My dearest Suze,

This in the greatest haste. I've been working on this paper for three days and was up at 4:30 a.m. to finish it. I just rolled it off the Xerox to take it home, pack and leave tomorrow at 8:00 a.m.

Big question, big favor to ask you. Could you do some editing on it? At least see if it makes sense the way I wrote it. I would be very grateful for your comments. Send your fax number.

Love you, Darling

Forever, your Da

"Look, there's a huge gap here. No letters since 1984 until this one in '88. Didn't Matthew die in '85? There must be a lot of letters from that time."

A SEASON OF MISTS

"Maybe they stopped keeping the letters for a period of time, or maybe they're in some other place. They didn't stop corresponding because this last letter is about Cora's prognosis, asking your mom not to call or write."

"Let me read it," Ellie says. "About that time, they decided to stop going back and forth about whether to stay together in some fashion. Belle Haven played a role, and they settled to take what time they could find."

Dec. 2, 1988

>Suze,
>
>My heart is heavy. Ominous black clouds are moving in, the air and humidity is stifling, and I feel as if I am trapped in a horrible, thorny, tropical jungle. I will call your office today.
>
>Cora has been diagnosed with pancreatic cancer. There's a procedure/surgery called the Whipple that might have delayed her death, but she has decided against it. She is being very brave. The doctors have told us approximately three months. The days slip by. My Darling, Suze, I am taking a three-month leave of absence in order to be absolutely available to her.
>
>Your Da
>
>P.S. Please don't write to the P.O. box or call the office. It will be hell, but I must let you go out of my life.

"That's the last of them. There aren't any letters after he tells her of Cora's disease. I know they corresponded after that, but when they began again or during that time, we've nothing. He must have gone through a kind of hell. He mentions that period in the letter she found on her bed the first night she returned to sleep in their bedroom. We lost Matthew in 1985. They each had hell to go through." Ellie says.

Maddy turns the last page. She sees Cora's name on the bottom of a typed page with a somewhat wobbly signature.

"Listen, Ellie, evidently before she became too sick, Cora wrote a letter to the children. Da must have tucked it into the box with the other letters. Her handwriting doesn't compare to Da's. It's cramped and more like printing.

"He must have found it after she died and never given it to them."

Dear Mary, Maureen, Paul and Phillip,

Before I'm no longer able to write a few words, I wanted to write this for you children and the grandchildren. You have a heritage that you won't understand until after I leave. We are Jews who suffered through the Holocaust (I will leave it up to your parents how much you want to tell your beautiful children: Dustin, Casey, Corrie, Daan and Charlotte).

Now before I die, I want to say what I've always felt too afraid to say: We are Jewish. I was a teenage wartime Dutch Resistance operative, and I helped hide nearly 100 Jews from the Germans during WWII. I forged identification papers for about eight dozen others.

I want to tell you one of my most poignant memories. It was 1940. I recall it easily. The Germans had invaded our homeland. I was dressed in a stolen nurse's uniform, making my way to Amsterdam's Central Station. I had received word that my father's youngest sister and three cousins were passing through on the way to Westerbork, the Nazi detention center in northeast Holland. My uncle had already been seized by the Nazis.

When I found my relatives in a railcar and knowing their destination, I asked if I could take my small cousin, a boy, about two years of age. I had him in my arms. The station was teeming with German soldiers, and I was stopped and questioned. I was so frightened I soiled my underwear. They could see I was an impostor and ripped the hat from my head. My dark hair came loose.

A SEASON OF MISTS

I had a false medical identification. I can't forget that moment of horror and fear. After slapping me about, they released me with our Adrian, someone you've known as your uncle. By then the trains were loaded, the whistles were blowing, the engines gasping, chuffing and pulsing more and more quickly, beginning that fateful trip trundling down the tracks.

Not too long after, the next day, when most of the soldiers had left, I bicycled to my uncle's farm to search for clothing for Adrian and to look after the animals. It was then I helped your father hide in the countryside on the farm. I bicycled and took him food without being caught.

I served as a messenger for the Underground movement, and helped publish a newspaper of Allied Forces' activities on a banned mimeograph machine. By taking it to him secretly, he was able to keep up to date and remain hidden.

Even though I am Jewish, I didn't have to wear a star. My father paid heavily for that. I was eighteen in 1940 when the Germans invaded. Life became more and more difficult for Jews. I never knew who was gone or who was in hiding. My whole life has been influenced by what happened in the war. I still have nightmares recalling that time. My whole family died eventually, including my parents and Adrian. By 1947, only 14,346 Jews remained in the Netherlands. Before the invasion there were 154,887.

Later, I learned that only about five percent of Dutch Jews survived. If you visit Westerbork, you'll see a red stone step for each life exterminated. Most were gassed upon arrival at concentration camps throughout Europe.

I have never been as brave as I was then. Now, I know that I am one of the last voices, and that I have been afraid and wrongly quiet since that time. All my father's brothers and sisters were gassed. Eventually, my father was unable to bribe his way out of predicaments, and both my parents were executed. Adrian was sent to an orphanage. Your father and I found records that referred to his death – more than likely from starvation.

I raised you children as Catholics even though Judaism is your heritage. I was afraid to give you your heritage. There's more to tell, but I am so tired just now. This should be more coherent. Your father doesn't agree with me that you should be told about my activities during the war. We have kept it private. One never knows who the enemy is. There are some things he doesn't know. For years, I never had to own my Judaism.

I've been afraid to this day to admit that I am a Jew. Your father and I contribute to the Holocaust Museum here in Washington, but I have never been. I couldn't have borne being reminded of the loss. We do not talk of those days. Continue to support this important effort, wherever you can, and speak out, out of respect for all who were lost to us.

I want you children to know these kinds of atrocities should never be allowed to happen again. Be honorable and brave in all you do. It's too late for me to speak out. I'm sorry I have stayed hidden to you. I believed I was protecting you.

Ellie lifts her head from Maddy's lap.

"Whew," Maddy says. Do you think your mother has read this?"

"I think she would have told us, don't you, about Cora, someone who suffered in silence, someone so heroic? Da told Mom that Cora was a recluse and felt afraid most of the time when she left the house alone. Da must have left this letter on the very bottom for your mom to find someday, or maybe never. I wonder why? Perhaps to explain his inability to leave Cora."

"Cora must have felt so damaged and haunted all those years by her memories. Not even Da could help her back."

"Maddy, I feel as torn as Da was." Ellie puts her head in her hands. "Had she known the pain Cora was in, I don't think Mom would have agreed to meet

Da all that time… if Cora saved his life. How could she have expected him to leave someone who saved his life? Their shared history is a powerful bond, the war, the children and all."

"You can choose not to tell her, Ellie. Simply remove the one letter written by Cora. It's more than eleven years ago. Your mom's in enough pain as it is. Da owed Cora his life, literally. That fact would hit her hard. Right now, she needs to heal. We don't want anything to detract from her memories of him. The illusion of their love keeps her alive.

"Realistically, Cora and Da probably never met the other's needs. Now isn't a good time for your mom to see this. They fell into being together because of the war, and then Cora became pregnant." Maddy feels out of her depth as a psychologist. She has always believed the truth was the best path, and here she is, advising against it.

"I really think Mom would have been sympathetic toward Cora, had she known how she suffered. She would have left Da.

"Coming out of Holland together as they did, Da must have meant the world to Cora. Surely, the intactness and security of their family meant everything to her. For Da, it must have been like paying a debt to Cora, not to leave her. Besides, it would have destroyed the family and would destroy the family now if they knew about Da's love for Mom before their mother died, especially if they were to learn of Mom and Da's long history."

"Finally, when she's dying, she comes out of hiding. She was quiet for over thirty-five years, and here in this simple note she wants to tell them her history and encourage them to be aware of the chance a similar pogrom could happen again. Why didn't Da pass it along?"

"I'm not sure. If the children don't know their mother's history and we gave it to them, I'm sure they'd begin to explore further and refer to it when together, like here at Belle Haven. It would be a huge topic among them. Mom would eventually find out that Cora was a survivor and a heroine in her time, the one who saved Da's life."

"For now, Ellie, let's keep it between us. I don't know what else to do."

"Maddy, I'm burning it."

Maddy meant to prevent her, but the flame began licking the curling edges and the letter was eaten by fire like the records of her family. Daan had to have been some compensation for her staggering losses.

Closing the cove

They rise late, except for Suzan. Suzan is at her easel concentrating, a brush in her hand. She has practically finished a weak sun rising through the shore pines and red alder from the vantage point of Bell Haven's driveway. *In this morning's sunrise, through the aureole of the crisp, cold light of fall, she's finding beauty in a new day,* Ellie thinks when she finds her. She has painted the scene with a little brown winter wren among the branches of a spindly pine. The bareness of the ground beneath is akin to the color of the wren.

At breakfast, Ellie complains that the substitute omelet pan is not as good as Da's, the one Mary took. Nonetheless, she succeeds at serving up two steaming, herb and cheese-laced omelets. Ellie and Suzan share. Maddy has mostly finished the speckled yellow crescent and says, "It just needs breaking in, El. Next time we're here, it'll be all seasoned."

"Mom, shall we come for Thanksgiving? You can meet Matthew. He'll be four months by then, unless you'd like to come to San Francisco?"

"Oh, Ellie, come here if you can."

Maddy and Ellie leave early on a bright morning. Ellie will drive her rental through the timbered, twisting curves to Portland, and Maddy will follow. Then they will head for S.F. on Interstate 5.

"Suzan, you're painting. I think I see a different style. Will you be taking them down to the gallery? People who know your work will see the difference too. Don't sell the one where you filled in the cove with that huge rock. I think you've given Da a symbolic tombstone."

Suzan waves to the backs of their cars. An arm out the window, they wave back. "We'll see you at Thanksgiving!"

A SEASON OF MISTS

Suzan goes to the porch out of habit to watch the ocean as she adjusts to the magnitude of the quiet. Even though it's cool, she opens a window to hear the sighs and sobs of the water. She's alone now with her loss, carrying her grief like a millstone, alone with the paralyzing, daily grind of grieving.

Maddy has left a colorful wool scarf on one of the leather chairs. Suzan toys with it, her thoughts turning to Ellie and Maddy, believing in them as a couple. Ellie seems to laugh more often. Maddy has a mothering quality, and for all her robustness, she can be quiet and reflective. And wise. *She's wise for her age,* Suzan thinks. *They'll be good parents.*

Suzan looks back to the rock that overhangs the cove, a tombstone from nature itself. She says 'yes' aloud. She turns quickly and carefully takes her still wet painting of the cove with the imagined displaced rock. She grabs a light jacket. For the first time since Da has gone, she drives, taking the Cadillac out. Da's driving glasses are in the seat, and she can smell his cologne. He loved this car, his third Cadillac. She raises the seat and stores the glasses. Later, when she sells the oversized car, she'll take them out and put them with all his other reading glasses she has collected around the house. His only clutter: his glasses and his books.

Maybe Frank is at the docks, in from his first run. She circles the lot and sees his charter boat. She parks and walks down the metal incline onto the wooden dock. She hears a pileated woodpecker at work on a piling. Bonaparte gulls swerve around her, shifting about and screeching. They flutter noisily and follow her as she walks farther. Among the schooners, charters and privately-owned fishing boats, among the masts and ropes, she finds him. The sea gently sloshes against the creaking dock.

Frank is a potential painting standing as he is, straddle legged, one foot on the dock, the other on his boat: his face, made red by the sun, the sea, the wind, all the elements, tell his story. His neck and arms, and his white beard trimmed at sharp angles expand on his story of devotion to all things nautical.

The area below his lower lip is cleanly shaved in a straight line just below his mustache. His smile below the purple, pocked nose deepens the ruts in his forehead. His muscles bulge through his shirt, and Suzan can see the whiteness of his skin where he has rolled his sleeves just beyond the faded tattoo of an anchor. A Navy man. She's never seen him without his captain's hat, but a lock of white hair has fallen onto his forehead. The boat is pristine. Her artist eyes take him in, surrounded by ropes and sails and flags.

He stoops, making a knot. Looking up, he sees her slimness through her jacket as she holds her arms wrapped around herself. He sees her anguished face.

"Oh, Frank!" she cries. "Da's gone. He's *gone!*"

Lashing a rope to the pier, he comes to her, and she seems fragile to him. She carries a scent of lavender.

She smells the fish on him, tangy and acrid, and her eyes brim with tears. He's silent, simply, clumsily flattening her hair, holding her head hard against his chest, and his scent is like the freshly caught fish, like the sea itself. She hears the gulls flapping as they settle again, closer to the catch. She hears the water slapping the sides of the boats. She sees a fisherman with a long green hose rinsing down his vessel. No wonder this setting filled Da's senses and lured him back.

The breeze transports the odor of the creosote from the pilings and the smell of the exhaust of diesel fuel. An inboard motor turns over and she feels the noise of the underwater churning in her chest.

"He was a fine man, Suzan. We've lost a fine man," Frank finally says in a gruff voice. Releasing her, he pulls out a handkerchief from his back pocket and blows his nose loudly, reminding Suzan of the foghorns. Unexpectedly she grins, and the submerged pain is cut back just as the vessel goes into gear and eases away from its mooring. The other more quiet sounds of the gulls skating above and about return.

"Frank, do you know where he died, in that smallest cove, just below us?"

Frank nods, "Yes, I know just the spot. He used to fish there. Favorite spot."

"There's a rock just above it, Frank. I want to move it and close up the cove where he died. Can you help me do it? I want to put a bench just above where the rock is now. I can already walk out on the sandstone and shale to that spot, but I'll make a stone path. Can you help me find the right people?"

"Wait a minute. You want to push that rock off into the cove? That's a mighty big rock." He says.

"I'll show you what I mean."

Suzan returns to the car and slides out the still-wet oil canvas of the rock painted as if nestled into the cove. She also has a photograph of where the rock, like a puzzle piece, sits now. The shape of it is like a huge deflated ball, caved in on the side toward the house, but projecting over the cove. The height and the flatness of the shelf make it an inviting spot to stand and watch the sea and judge the tide.

"I see what you mean, Suze. It looks like a perfect fit. The trick would be to get her to land just so." He calls her Suze, just like Da. His roughened hand is on his forehead. He pushes his cap back and resettles it. Suzan can see that the bright red skin doesn't extend beyond the neckline of his tee-shirt. Her heart is softened by the rubescent weathered captain. "Frank, I feel so lost," she says.

"It'll be that way for a while. My Eloise went quickly like that."

"Suze, let me talk to my crew. I'll ask a couple of lumberjacks. They're always moving big equipment and stuff. By golly, I think we can do it. I have an old spruce mast that might work to pry it off there, if I cut her down a little. Need something long and strong, a fulcrum and some muscle, maybe a couple of crowbars. The boys and me, we'll come by and take a look. What the heck kind of a job for a fisherman?"

He's touched by her idea and needs to think it through. He thought a lot of Daan, Da, she calls him. They were good together, those two. They were good for the community too, him working on the school board and all.

Frank signals for her to wait a minute. He steps onto his charter boat, named for his deceased wife Eloise. Toward the back she sees him whack off the head of a Chinook salmon. Another whack and he holds up a piece of red-fleshed fish, its skin glistening like engraved polished silver, shrugging his broad shoulders as if it's a question.

"Yes," she says to his unvoiced question as she cups her hands against her mouth. "I'll have it this evening."

"Nothing like it," he says. "Will you be home tomorrow afternoon? We'll be by – Earl, me and Tom. I have to take a bunch of doctors out in the morning. Seems like I always get one who gets seasick."

Suzan stops by Samantha's By the Sea Gallery even though it's early. A For Sale sign is newly posted outside. Surprised, she parks in the gravel lot, which is slowly being taken over by grass and dandelions, and goes to the door, her painting in hand. Samantha stands surveying the back wall of paintings, her hands on her square hips. Her graying hair is gathered rather carelessly to the back. Her clothes are loose and flowing, long to her ankles, and increase the perception that she is a large woman. By the gray in her long coarse hair, she is perhaps sixty years old. She has been a friend. Suzan knocks lightly.

Samantha pushes Suzan away at arm's length, her hands on Suzan's shoulders and looks her in the face. "I'm so sorry, Suzan. I know his family came. Will there be a service? None of us have heard."

Samantha lives in a spacious studio apartment above the gallery. A large gray cat wanders down the pine stairway, tail waving slowly, coming to Suzan and brushing against her leg. As the cat comes back for another rub, back arched, Suzan stoops to run her hand along his back. "How are you, Sooty?"

Looking up to Samantha, she says, "How can you be selling, Samantha? You've been here for twenty-five years! This is your dream. You have that wonderful studio upstairs beside this one where you teach. This is any artist's dream. There's good traffic, even in the winter."

"Mother needs my help," she states. "She's had a stroke, and I have to get her placed in a home. I'll just have to find my way from there, because no matter what, I'll need to be near her. Seattle is just too far away to try and manage what looks like expensive long-term care, hopefully in her own home."

"I'm sorry, Samantha. You must be overwhelmed."

"With these stairs, she can't come here, even if she succeeds at rehab. There aren't any long-term facilities around here. Besides, the gallery takes up nearly all my time. She may regain some use of her left arm. Her speech is affected. That's the hardest part, communicating with her, Suzan, plus I'm the only one there for her. I think she understands what I say, but I have my work cut out for me. At eighty-five, she can improve only so much."

"It'll be a long, hard time, coming back from a stroke," Suzan says.

"If I sell, I can buy some time to get the situation resolved. I'll also need the money. They want to dismiss her from the hospital, but they haven't found space in a suitable rehab center. The social workers are working on it every day, and we may have a lead on an opening coming up next week. She has just enough money; we'll have to pay for her care. I don't want to sell her home. My brothers won't be of any help. They are barely making it now."

"Medicare won't pay?"

"Not yet, not until we drain her resources. Could you stand in for me here? You'd have to let the realtors bring their clients."

"Certainly, I can. But, I'll be so sorry to see you sell. Shall I take my paintings out?"

"I think your paintings will sell before it goes to another owner. You've developed quite a reputation."

Samantha draws in a deep breath and blows it out. "Suzan, if you really could run the gallery for a couple of weeks until I get things settled for Mother, it would be such a help. I'd like you to stay here in the apartment. I know you're hurting up there all alone."

"Yes, Samantha. I can do it."

"Can Sooty stay? She has her own habits, likes to be outdoors in the afternoon. She always comes home to the back door. You'll find her sitting there about five o'clock."

"Sure, Sooty can stay, although I've not had much experience with cats. I just need to be home a few days before Thanksgiving. Paul and his family are coming, so is Ellie. I'm planning a small memorial service for Daan. I'd like for you to come."

"I should be back a week or so before then. Today, I need to get the paperwork ready for the realtor to show that I've had a profit these years. What is it, mid-October? I'll be back in plenty of time. I'm glad it's a slower time of the year."

Suzan shows Samantha her painting. "This isn't for sale, but I thought it might be nice in the window. Samantha, this is where he died. I've painted the rock above it into the cove. In my imagination, I closed the cove."

Suzan turns the canvas so it faces Samantha. "The grays and blues are beautiful, Suzan. How do you capture them? They're in your head, that's all. I wish I had your gift for catching the light. It's perfect for the window. It'll draw people in. It's a larger canvas than you usually use."

"May I paint in the back studio while I'm here, back where you teach?"

"Of course. You could give some lessons yourself. Why not take over my students? There are only three."

"When would you want me to begin?"

"I'd like to leave here by Monday morning. I don't want them to move her without my being there. In the meantime, I'll be making calls."

"Just be in touch, and leave lots of instructions."

Suzan stops by to see Rosie. "Good morning darling, Suzan. I've been on my knees for you, and here you are as pretty as a picture. Ellie, too. I don't think she eats much of what she buys; she's skinny as a rail. Could be in a magazine, you two. He was a real gentleman, Suzan. We're all missing him. The morning Frank came in here telling me, I gave him two dozen donuts for those boys on his boat. They've all got to be sad. Da did like his fishing be it from his cove or out with Frank."

"Rosie, would you be able to organize some food for a small memorial reception for Da?"

"Darling, I'd do anything for you. You poor, dear thing. If it's not a weekend, I can do anything. Let's sit a minute."

Rosie pours Suzan's favorite dark roast, fluffs her white apron in front of her and sits, with hands folded as if she has all morning long to talk. Suzan reaches for the cream from another table.

"Rosie, I want to move that big rock above the cove where Da died down into the cove where he was standing the moment it happened. We'll do it Thanksgiving morning, when its high tide, as close to dawn as possible. I'll have to check my tide book. After that I want to serve up a memorial reception for his friends. Ellie and her friend are coming. Would Thanksgiving morning close to dawn work for you? You're welcome to stay for dinner later."

"Well, I'll be. That's a new idea. It's a good one, sweetheart. I'll be closed all that day. The ones who haven't gotten their pies for the big day, it'll be too late for them. I'll be at Belle Haven any time of day you want me," Rosie says. "I've seen those two girls together. They're a real pair. That Maddy can keep up Ellie's spirits. She lost somebody pretty special too."

Belle haven

Suzan stops at the end of the drive to pick up the mail. Paul's letter is succinct and direct:

> I'm writing with regard to Belle Haven. As you know my father and I were investment partners in the dairy company, Dairico, here in Denver that I founded. Dad's investments have paid off very well. Dairico is thriving and expanding. (We now have 3,000 cows in each of the four locations.)
>
> Just after you married, Dad bought Belle Haven out of his investment in Dairico. We agreed to put the title in Dairico's name, so Belle Haven is essentially owned by the company. As the will says, you inherit everything except the investment in Dairico. I'm assuming you know all this, but I wanted to tell you.
>
> I feel strongly about leasing Belle Haven by the week, beginning this spring, as a vacation house. Phillip and I have looked into what's available to tourists in comparison to Belle Haven. There's not much. There's a waiting list, and those that are available to rent year-round are few. Belle Haven would be a good income resource. Whichever direction we go, you should probably plan to be moved by early June.

Paul has enclosed a written copy of both the eulogy Da's brother, Jaan, gave and the obituary. She sets them aside to read later, but notes immediately that Suzan Vandivere is not listed as the surviving wife but that Da was preceded in death by Cora Vandivere, his wife of over thirty-seven years. It's as if Suzan didn't exist. *I've been written out,* she thinks.

Suzan calls Paul immediately after reading the letter. After a series of transfers through receptionists and assistants, she speaks with him directly. Suzan's voice is shaky early in the conversation. But, she regains her posture and states strongly, "I didn't know this information, and I want to continue to live here. It's my home."

"Obviously, Dad didn't intend for you to live on at Belle Haven or he would have set it up differently. As it stands now, the house belongs to Dairico."

"But it was your father's intent that I should continue to live at Belle Haven, that it would become mine."

"Dad never told me of those intentions. I'd honor them if he had, but he didn't."

After saying goodbye, Suzan holds on to the back of a chair, trembling, trying to control her fear, her anger. She needs relief from the shock of her compounded loss. She calls Ellie, but Ellie's phone goes to the message service.

She calls their financial advisor, Rex.

"Rex, there's enough in the estate to buy back Belle Haven. Da wanted it to be mine."

"You'd be broke thereafter. First off, they're not obligated under the law to sell it to you. Can you prove it was his intent?"

"But he meant for me to have Belle Haven. He mentions it even in his last letter to me. I can prove it, but the letter would break us all apart. I want to buy Belle Haven if that's necessary."

"You need an attorney, Suzan, to somehow prove his intention that it was to go to you. That's unfinished business on Da's part."

"Rex, I can't use the letter to prove his intent. It reveals other personal information that the family shouldn't know."

Suzan will have to choose between keeping Belle Haven and disclosing Da's and her long-term relationship, ending forever the legacy Da meant to leave his family. All would be revealed, and she would lose them as family forever.

"Suzan, take what you have and see Tom Kinkaid here in town. Take all the paperwork you can dig up. Show him your check to Da when you bought the house. Evidently, Da put that money into Dairico. See what he can tell you. Paul, as CEO, and Da must have had a lease agreement so the two of you could continue to live there even though the deed is in Dairico's name. I'm sorry Suzan, it's a mess."

"I don't understand, I thought Belle Haven was mine. I knew nothing about it being tied up with Dairico. I knew nothing about a lease."

Suzan knows for certain now, that she will permanently alter the cove. She doesn't want the strangers who might live here seeing or using the cove where he died. Without Da, without Belle Haven, where will she make a home?

In the same batch of mail are two unevenly folded pictures from Corrie, pictures of Suzan. In one her mouth is turned down. It's a gray, rainy day. The rain is heaviest over her head. In the other, in bright sunlight, Suzan smiles. Suzan smooths them flat against the table. On each picture, a pink heart is drawn in, just above Corrie's signature.

That evening, when the light is retreating, the atmosphere dyeing the sky a deep purple, Teri calls to check on Suzan. Obviously, Paul hasn't told her of his call or the letter.

"How are you doing? Is it going better? I know you miss him terribly. We all do. I can just see him slipping his arm around you."

Suzan doesn't let on that she knows she may lose Belle Haven. Instead, she says, "Oh, Teri. It's great of you to call. After everyone left I hardly knew what to do. The house is so empty without him. We loved it here together. Ellie and Maddy, whom you haven't met, are partners now, and they'll be here for Thanksgiving. They've been cleared to adopt a little baby boy. It will be quite a family celebration."

"I'm so happy for you. Suzan," Teri says. "Daan and Charlotte want to come to Belle Haven again, and see where their grandfather died. They have many wonderful memories of Belle Haven and their grandfather."

"Why don't you and the family come for Thanksgiving?"

"Let me talk with Paul. It might be the perfect time with the long weekend. Of all things, young Daan is interested in Marine Biology and thinks the University of Oregon would be a good school for him. He's already applied."

It's three o'clock the next day when Frank, Earl and Bob pull up. Suzan has coffee ready. Together, mugs in their hands, they walk down the slight slope of shale layers toward the top of the cove. Earl hands his mug to Bob and leaps down inside the cove. "Looks pretty near ready to slide on in," he says, shouting against the wind and the breaking waves.

Bob has knelt beside the rock, scraping with his hands around it. "Some of these rocks can be dug out from underneath to help her slide. We can pulverize some of these larger ones or just move them beforehand."

Frank steps off what he thinks the length the mast will need to be. "I'll be durned, I think it's about perfect the way it is. We'll need a couple more fellas to help pull her down. Son of a bitch, I think we got it figured out," he talks aloud to himself.

He walks back to Suzan, who has gathered the mugs on a rock beside her. He grins, and the facial muscles of a man who has seen more sun than shade contract into a ready smile, deepening the wrinkles across his brow, closing up the white creases around his eyes.

A white four-wheel drive truck, its tires larger than normal, pulls up. They can hear the exhaust even as it idles. Suzan and Frank go out front to meet them. "Sorry we're a little bit late. We got to talking about our next cutting job, and time just got away from us, that's all." Johnny says. He and Gus both dismount, greeting Suzan with a lift of their caps.

"Here's my muscle, Suze, meet Gus and Johnny."

"What do you have here, man?" Johnny asks.

"A little taste of hell, that's what," Frank says

Before noon they have a plan. She leaves them be and watches from the window. They slap each other lightly on the shoulder and walk toward their trucks.

She steps outside where their trucks are parked. "We'll need one of your big rigs to get that mast over here," She hears Frank shout to Johnny.

"Not a problem, we'll have her here when you need her. We'll have a winch too. Hey, you got anything left over from the catch this morning?"

"You bet I do. Come on by and have a look at that mast while you're at it. You realize you have to bring it back down to the dock yard. Can't leave it here unless Suzan wants to buy a flag pole."

Frank and his boys squeeze into the cab of the Ford pickup. "Let me figure the time for high tide that morning," he says to Suzan, leaning out the window.

That evening Ellie and Maddy call, each on the phone at the same time. "Mom, he gets to come home earlier than they expected. He's beautiful. His hair is nearly white, and he has the bluest eyes."

"I've taken two weeks off as maternity leave. Ellie will take the next two, and we'll all be up for Thanksgiving weekend."

"Is little Matt sleeping through the night?" Suzan asks.

When they have asked and answered all the questions about Matt, Suzan tells them of Paul's letter and their conversation by phone. "Wow, I never dreamed…" Ellie says. "How are you going to fight it? Do you have a plan? We all know Da wanted you to have Belle Haven."

"I have some time. Right now, I'm planning a memorial service for Da at dawn Thanksgiving morning." Suzan credits Maddy for the idea of moving the rock. "Now it's coming about. Frank wants to take the Eloise out with the family to fish when it's over. We can stay back with Matthew and prepare Thanksgiving dinner."

"Mom, maybe I'll ask around a bit for a lawyer here in San Francisco. There's got to be a way to keep Belle Haven without disclosing your history with Da."

Suzan tells them of her plans to cover for Samantha at the gallery. "It's for sale, Ellie."

Hanging up, Suzan reads the obituary. One can know by reading it in the *Washington Post* that he was a successful man, a lover and patron of the arts, a person with many interests and strong family ties. He was a landscape artist, a gardener. She enjoyed that he tediously tended his roses and orchids, varieties of which he picked up on his many trips all over the world with the World Bank. Years before, he had told her of the several orchids from Singapore that sat in his office window and thrived despite those sometimes brutal winters in D.C. She must learn how to care for those he's left.

He was a pianist, a student of several languages (that with his strong Dutch accent, gave him a worldliness that aroused her affection for him). He became a Catholic on American shores. The obituary says a mass was held October 6, 2000, four days after his death. Da's brother, Jaan, ten years his junior gave a lengthy eulogy, telling those present no one had known him in full. Da had confided in him about his love for Suzan and corresponded with him often.

Daan had pursued a double doctorate in agronomy and statistics, finishing his long career at the World Bank, in Washington, D.C. Prior to his career at the World Bank, he owned a business based in Sacramento in the early 70's, near the campus of the university. He was hired subsequently by the World Bank and came to Washington as project manager for various agricultural endeavors funded by the World Bank around the world.

She continues to read Jaan's handwritten eulogy:

One could say, in a sense, he was an accomplished Renaissance man. Father of four, he had a long marriage to Cora. Da was a patron of the arts, a ten-year board member of the Bach Festival in Eugene, Oregon, a supporter of the Opera League in Portland, Oregon, a volunteer at a local homeless shelter, a Master Gardener with the University of Oregon and a teacher in Lincoln City, Oregon Community Literary Council. He embraced life with extraordinary passion and love. He was an artist, oil painter, gardener, and pianist. He was proficient in many languages and a serious student of philosophy, religion, and culture. But, most importantly, he passionately loved and respected his wife, family, and friends. He was a gentleman's gentleman.

Daan was born in Java, Indonesia. His family moved back to their native Netherlands shortly after. He graduated from high school as the Nazis invaded in 1940. He spent the war years at the university and in hiding after escaping "labor camp". It was his wife who helped him gain entry to the University in Amsterdam. Cora was from a prominent Jewish family. Following the war, Daan continued his studies at the University of Wageningen, Netherlands, earning his Masters in Tropical Agronomy and his professional engineering designation. He was awarded a scholarship to attend Iowa State University where he obtained a Masters in Soil Fertility and Plant Pathology.

My brother, Dr. Vandivere, began his career in Malaysia as a Research Botanist and Rubber Plantation Manager. Later, he returned to the United States to earn his Ph.D. in Agronomy as well as Statistics. During an assignment in Hawaii, he solved a technical pineapple problem. He launched his career as an

American citizen as an international agriculture development expert with an interlude as a research scientist. He and his family celebrated the Statehood of Hawaii by becoming Naturalized American citizens.

He worked at senior levels in more than sixty countries for public and private entities. Along the way, he took his family to live in Africa, Asia, and Europe. His significant projects assisted many third world countries gain some self-sufficiency in food production, helping make true his dream of eliminating hunger world-wide.

Suzan places the copy of the eulogy beside her bed to read again. Suze loved attending the summertime Bach Festival, with more than forty events from which to choose. The programs offered Monteverdi, Verdi, Bach, Rachmaninoff, Mozart, Milhaud and many others. There were workshops, seminars, free community events. Da was tireless. They had found a lodge on the McKenzie River, which welcomed them every year as they indulged up to their ears.

Suzan knows Cora was a Jewess, who fled with him to America in the mid 40's. He was hiding out, secretly tilling the tidelands for vegetables beneath the dikes before they met, while the world reeled, the rumors swirled, and the Nazis prevailed, and were apt to send the likes of him to labor camps or just kill a man outright.

The eulogy doesn't tell the whole story, but she tries to fill in with what he has told her. She doesn't know that Ellie and Maddy have discovered Cora's letter and know even more than she does. She doesn't know that Cora was an underground operative who saved Da's life. She doesn't know that Paul was conceived before he and Cora married. She doesn't know that the reason for his inability to leave Cora was his lifetime indebtedness to her, and a commitment at seventeen for having impregnated her.

Food and water

1940 Amsterdam

When Cora wrote to her children about her role in the Resistance Movement, she didn't tell them that before she got home that day with baby Adrian, the same two soldiers followed her, and both raped her without regard inside the women's restroom. They first removed her soggy underpants. One soldier held Adrian who was screaming while the other raped her. She dug her fingernails into the arms of the first and scratched the face of the second.

She cried out for help. By then the trains were loaded, the whistles were blowing and there was no one to hear or to help her. The sounds of the chuffing train, the steam escaping, stayed with her until her death. She never again used a kettle to boil water because the hiss of the steam and the whistle reminded her of the harm done her and to her entire family.

She was raped because she looked Jewish. They said that her features betrayed her, making fun especially of her nose; it was too prominent to be otherwise. They tore up her fake identification. The soldiers were young and swaggered out of the restroom leaving her on the cement floor with Adrian squalling beside her.

She washed and washed, removing the skin and blood under her nails, scrubbing herself with lye soap even when it hurt her to do so. She lay sick in bed for a full day. Her mother, believing it was time for her cycle, brought hot tea and toast. Her mother knew Cora often experienced premenstrual cramping and paid little attention.

Cora woke, crying out in the night. Her mother was occupied with little Adrian, who suffered from fear of the dark. Her cries were unheard. The

Of Unseen Things Above

Myrna L Brown
Author

817 Fox Ridge Lane
Wilmington, North Carolina

910-509-0112
mrsmlbrown@ec.rr.com

nightmares would overtake her sleep life, and she would never recover because after that night, other horrors were added to her memories. She would lose her entire family to venomous hate and lust.

The following morning, her father was visibly distraught. His hands shook as he held the sleeping child on his shoulder. At his request, she bicycled painfully to her uncle's farm to search for clothing for Adrian and to look after the animals, the unfed calves and the unmilked cows sure to be swollen and suffering. As she pedaled in on the tracks through the grass of the drive, she could hear the calves bawling in the barn.

The hinges of the screen creaked as she carefully opened the farmhouse door. Immediately, she gagged, and the stagnant smells released from the warm kitchen caused her to go to the yard and vomit. The table was covered with thick, blackened blood where the raiding German soldiers had butchered part of a milk cow. Pots, partially filled with putrid stew were still on the stove. The disturbed flies buzzed about, landing again on the feast of rot. Otherwise there was complete silence. Smashed pottery lay about. She picked up a tea cup, but the saucer had broken. She held her apron against her face and stepped across the room.

Upstairs she found the few blankets left behind strewn on the floor. The windows were open. The rain had blown in, and the starched, white curtains were soiled and droopy. Instinctively, she closed the windows, locking the sashes.

She checked on the remaining animals. The bloated carcasses of the three Guernsey milk cows, killed at close range with the Germans' pistols, their legs stiff in the air, lay near the entrance to the loft. One cow had been partially butchered; its ribs were exposed. The entrails had puddled and were beginning to shrink from exposure. Their slobber as they died had rimmed about their lips, white and ghostly. Blood had trickled through their nostrils.

Going inside the barn, the calves butted the pen and crowded each other. They stretched their necks, bleating as only distraught calves do, crowding toward her. She pumped water and brought it to them one by one. She released them to the pasture where she hoped they'd find nourishment and water even as young as they were. The nippled metal buckets from which they were milk fed were of no use now, but she hung them on the rail of the pen as if to restore some kind of order. They clanged together as she handled them, and the noise echoed in the empty barn. The dust the calves had stirred was caught by the little light there was as it filtered down through the semi-darkness onto Cora's hair. She began to climb the outside door to the loft to see if any hay had been put up for the winter. Perhaps the young calves would feed on it in desperation.

Daan, as he was always known to her, her cousin from a farm farther north lay in the hay quietly waiting when she started up the ladder. He had watched as she bicycled up the lane; he saw her enter and retreat quickly from the house to vomit. She re-entered, and he watched as she returned and tied a bundle of clothes into the basket on her bike. He could see she was fit, lean and long legged. Suddenly, he recognized her as Cora, his little cousin, grown up. "Cora, Cora," he whispered loudly, swinging open the hayloft door.

"Daan, they didn't find you?" she said when she discovered him.

"I was bringing word from my father about the rumors he'd heard. I was too late, and hid beneath the hay. I could hear the sobs and the anguish of the family. I lay there while they were here, then all night and yet another day after they left. They killed all three cows. They released the rabbits and took down the chicken wire. They took the whole family as prisoners after making them cook one of the hens and part of the cow. I would be eating the eggs, but they've been smashed or taken."

"They took the family to Grand Station; they were stuffed in a rail car." She said. "I saved Adrian, the baby." Cora described everything except the rape.

Cora pulled her lunch from beneath her breast. "What have you been eating?"

"I've only had the water I was carrying. It's nearly finished."

Lying to her parents, she continued to come, bringing him food, sometimes not until late in the evening. Her parents knew she was part of the growing underground resistance and knew her to be out late. Her father had paid, and she didn't have to wear the star. She had also received new papers. She explained she had been roughed up trying to get to Adrian and they burned her ruined uniform.

Cora and Daan were young and began to explore and respond to each other very shyly. It began when he dropped part of the bread she brought onto the slatted floor of the loft. Squatting beside him, she brushed it off and put it very deliberately in his mouth. He caught her hand briefly.

They hadn't seen each other in two years. They felt newly introduced. They lay on their backs talking of the future, what might happen after the war. Surely it would end. They talked of their studies and the possibility of university for him. Sometimes, they talked of going to America. Daan continued to hide. Cora told him her father could be of influence. Papers could be forged.

Their hands touched as they lay together. Only narrow shafts of light came through the barn roof, and often it grew dark before they stopped talking. On such an evening, Cora waited until he fell asleep and crept up beside him to spend the night.

She lay close against him on the straw he had arranged as his bed, believing his gentle person could undo the harm done her, as if the brutality could be mitigated. She also knew she might have been impregnated by one of the soldiers because she hadn't had her monthly cycle.

Waking in the night, realizing she was there, he became aroused; he quickly raised her skirt and was atop her before she could fully waken. He expected she wanted him to find her and do just so. She had touched his erection through his trousers earlier that day. He had never touched her there. He barely knew his way into her vagina.

She cried, pushing him away while still clinging to him; she continued to resist, and they fumbled until he became exceedingly gentle and entered her again in a measured way, caressing her and leaving her clothes on. She didn't experience orgasm, nor would she ever. A great shame enveloped her. The anguish of the rapes interfered with any pleasure, even though she had healed and the bruises on her thighs had turned yellow. She couldn't show him how to please her, and he didn't know to do anything except hold her when she cried.

She continued to cry, even on subsequent nights, releasing herself to his physical advances until the moment she began to relive the trauma of the rapes. At seventeen, though he would never know, he had lost his virginity to a girl who had recently been raped by two German soldiers... a girl of eighteen.

The Netherlands was no longer neutral, but the resistance was slow to gain momentum. Again, she stole a uniform, that of an SS soldier. There was much confusion and multiple rank titles of the earthen gray service dress uniforms. She was able to move about almost freely, but still preferred evenings and nights. She brought him the undercover flyers they printed from a stolen mimeograph. The typographical errors were typed over and appeared darker, like tiny bullet holes on the thin, pink paper. As soon as he read them, they were torn into tiny bits and shoved under the straw like confetti.

She told him of her undercover activities, her false identities, those she helped fabricate and the people who counted on her to escape the camps. She helped hide those most at risk. Sometimes those in the underground didn't know who was hidden and who had been taken. She never told him of the harm done her.

They continued to touch. After their first experience, he was able to reach beneath her blouse and stroke her breasts. Her nipples stood to his touch, and he wished to see them. He smelled beneath her arms, smothering his face and stroked the smoothness of her inner thighs, but she let him go no farther with his hands, nor could he see. When they had intercourse, she cried as if she were lost. She wanted him and repelled him at the same time. Confused, he felt an obligation to be responsible for her and touched her face over and over to reassure her.

She waited for her monthly cycle, but it never came. Pregnant and frightened, she talked of Daan with her parents. Strings were pulled. He was able to enroll at the university. Living with her parents and Adrian, they had a child and named him Paul. Cora was relieved when Paul grew a healthy head of black hair. He was no Aryan. Even though her family would die by the hand of the Germans, she was saved.

Adrian was walking when he came to live with them. He walked everywhere looking for his mother inside the home and in the garden. When Cora and Daan's little Paul came, he was like a pet for Adrian, and Adrian was protective and attentive, even sitting beside Paul's crib as he slept. To Paul, Adrian became something like a brother.

Cora's wealthy father found them a way to America and supported them during Daan's schooling. Still making ends meet was difficult, and at one point Daan sold encyclopedias from door to door. Daan never released himself from being responsible for Cora's well-being, though she became closed to his affection. He didn't understand nor could he summon the will to love her.

Over the years, she resisted his efforts to bring her even the slightest pleasure, but stoically, she accepted him and bore him four children. Over the years, she hovered over her family, caring for them in tedious ways. She darned their socks and knit them sweaters. She studied about nutrition. Her children drank gallons of milk and ate their vegetables. Over the years, she measured and weighed the enriched bread she made even though they wanted white bread from the store. Everything had a place, and everything was in its place. She was not penurious but nearly so.

She focused on her children as they came along. She followed him in his career, from Hawaii, to Asia, to Africa and finally to the States. She was uninterested in Daan's attempts to woo her. He constructed a barrier, as impenetrable as hers, and they were withdrawn and quiet when alone together. "A world apart," he described it to Suze.

They worked hard that he might have a career in the field he loved. He was idealistic in his thinking that he could help change the world through agriculture. There should be no hunger, the numbers showed, he believed. The problem is one of distribution. He believed those who couldn't prosper were more prone to violence. To covet is to corrupt one's self and it seemed to him when the very poor lived amongst the wealthy and powerful, corruption prevailed.

The goal remains unachieved. Then again, perhaps he did change the future for many people through his efforts.

New haven

In the three weeks that have passed, their half a mountain in late afternoon light is transformed into varied tones of amber, ablaze in the setting sun as she drives home. She enters through the garage and stands before the great windows, sickened by the silence. She checks the tenebrous rooms as they shed their light and begin to chill, adjusting the thermostat or fluffing a pillow. She begins making lists, preparing for Thanksgiving Day. She returns to the less gloomy gallery.

Samantha's By the Sea Gallery sits on the corner of Main Street. Rosie's is in the middle of the block. The small parking lot beside the gallery is often used by Rosie's customers, coming and going. As people walk past, they sometimes stand at the windows, pointing and talking. While there, nothing of Da surrounds her, but she can imagine him coming through the door, unannounced, carrying coffee or bringing a canvas he has stretched for her.

Those who know of her loss come in to offer their sympathies, and she is reminded daily that Belle Haven sits cold and empty until she goes briefly in the evenings to retrieve the mail and check on things. Da is gone. There is no greater emptiness. She feels a need to be in both places, to sit with his absence there and be at the gallery.

Since Frank has offered to take Paul, Teri, Charlotte and young Daan out on his charter boat immediately after they move the memorial stone into the cove, Suzan will need to provide some kind of substantial snack and drinks. She'll need to pick up Dramamine to prevent seasickness. Ellie and Maddy will stay back with the baby and help prepare the turkey dinner. Rosie, too, is invited for dinner. With Frank, they'll be nine people. A twenty-pound turkey should do it. She calls Arthur and gives him the entire list.

A SEASON OF MISTS

Before she goes back to feed Sooty, she rereads her last letter from Da:

> Our reservations are made. I knew you would agree to Paris. I knew you would say yes. I'll take you to Le Tour for the best duck in the world. It's a famous restaurant that overlooks Notre Dame. We'll find Reubens' famous women at the Louvre (they remind me so of you). We'll walk the Champs. We'll be dazzled again by the Christmas lighting, the Eiffel Tower as it changes colors all night long. I wonder if that insightful old woman at that little apartment on Rue du Bac is still living. I'll take you to the café where first I wrote you, just near that church.

She is reminded that she must call United Airlines and the hotels to cancel their bookings for December. Her lists for herself are long, and her mind is healing as she encumbers herself with chores, or as she quietly describes an artist's background to a customer, offering ten percent off if the painting is sold that day.

The art has been selling well, and she rearranges the gallery. She brings more of her own in to fill the empty spots. Samantha has stopped the stream of new pieces coming from New York and Chicago.

The realtor brings in clients, dreamers usually, who want to live an ideal: own a little business, have a quiet life by the sea. He shows them the accounting books, noting that Samantha made a $75,000 profit last year. The current year is doing as well.

The wren appears again in her work, and her thoughts go often to Da who wooed her for so many years; who continued to woo her during these last years, even though she never once thought of leaving him. His song was varied and strong, sometimes repetitious if he needed to sing out his heart from some far place within himself. Sometimes, like the wren, several months would go by, and he would revisit his repertoire, the same words in the same rhythm. "I love you, I love you," he would repeat. She didn't tire of hearing him. It was his way.

In the morning the ethers of the paint, the smell of coffee, the array of art combine with the close company – Suzan's senses are filled. She loses track of time. On those days, Sooty reminds her at the back door when it's 5:00 p.m.

Teri calls the following day to tell Suzan of an eight-week internship in Marine Biology that will be held over the summer located at Coos Bay, about four hours down the coast. The eight-week term is available as well as several two-week and weekend workshops. The eight-week course aligns with young Daan's interest in Invertebrate Zoology, how they look, live and behave as well as their natural history and how near they are to extinction, which hasn't yet been established through research.

"There will be extensive field trips to rocky shores, estuaries as well as the sandy shoreline. Live animals will be available to study in the lab," she reads to Suzan.

Will she be here she wonders? Suzan remembers young Daan bringing in such specimens over the years when he spent his holidays here. When he was small, he even brought her the black tadpoles looking like swimming apple seeds, from a nearby pond, careful to keep them afloat by cupping both hands, one on top of the other. Da and he puzzled over the more unusual specimens he brought and tried to find references to a particular environment. How would they fare in the future, Da had asked of Daan. Who's going to protect them?

Grandfather and grandson, together shared interests that led them through many searches, and Suzan remembers Da talking with his namesake about the depth of the Mariana Trench in the Pacific, an incision nearly seven miles deep, the deepest part of the earth. He showed him where it was located near Guam, and they looked up a species peculiar to it. "In the cold and the darkness of its depth of nearly seven miles, the unusual fish are big, very wide and have fins that resemble wings. The tail is elongated like an eel and the face resembles the markings of a shell. The explorers nicknamed it the 'ghost fish' because its outer skin was nearly translucent," Daan had read aloud to his grandfather, one finger moving across and down as he stumbled on connecting some of the syllables.

All her memories, those most precious are tied to Da, to Da and Belle Haven, where it will always seem he is expected.

After Teri's call, Suze goes out of the drizzle and fog, into the gallery warm and snug. The art students come three days a week for the two weeks Suzan is there. Over the afternoons, they bond and tell their stories. Rusty's wife is gone now since three years. He has learned to cook for himself and often describes a newly discovered recipe. He seems to assume the widows have never sautéed or braised or marinated. It's still all new to him, being in the kitchen. He's portly and has a high energy level, often erupting if he is disappointed in his choice of colors or the stroke of his brush.

Unlike the robust, volatile Rusty, Da was trim and imperturbable, refined in his ways. By contrast, Suzan appreciates Da all the more. Even though he is gone, her affection for him increases. It is in one of these moments she might go upstairs and allow herself a moment of solitude, grabbing a tissue from the half-bath to dab her eyes.

Death isn't stalking her now; she is alert and has found her way out of its shadow; her ears are willfully closed to its taunts. Even in the absence of joy, she begins to understand she has entered a new phase of her life, a life without Da. She will never know Cora's history. She views her with envy, but without the compassion the truth may have compelled her to feel.

Young Daan applies for the internship in Marine Biology through the University of Oregon in Coos Bay. With his grades, level of activity and advanced placement classes, the turnaround is quick; he is accepted to be among a group of twenty others. He will be accepted into the university for the fall semester as well, Teri reports to Suzan.

"He very much wants to go out to Oregon to school. You should see how he pores over the information. Suzan, over these years I believe he fell in love with all things about the sea because of our time with you there in Belle Haven. Well, nature itself. He has no interest whatsoever in his father's dairy business. May he come there on the weekends this summer? When he goes to the university, can he use Belle Haven as home base? By the way, if the invitation is still open, we'll come there over the Thanksgiving weekend. We'd like to drive both to Coos Bay and Eugene to get a feel for things. Also, our teens want to see where their grandfather died."

"My goodness, yes. Come! Oh Teri, what does Paul think of Daan's ideas? What a wonderful opportunity to get hands-on experience even before he enters his freshman year. I think he already knows as much as they do."

June is the expected time for Suzan to leave Belle Haven. Paul must not have discussed the matter with Teri. All along, Teri assumes Suzan will be there. If Suzan were to tell of her long illicit history with Da she could prove his intentions, but the price is too high. Better to lose Belle Haven. There's a chest from China, rugs from Turkey, crystal from Sweden, a lithograph from

Amsterdam taken from the original copper etching by Rembrandt. The piano. What will she take? Where will she go?

Change of course

Ellie and Maddy's child is beautiful at nearly four months. Maddy has been up in the night and is getting some sleep while Ellie holds him in the morning light near the kitchen. Suzan is moving about in preparation for Thursday. The light glances off his nearly bald crown. Suzan comes to cradle his head in her hand before Ellie puts him down. His chest is rising and falling evenly. His one piece sleeper is soft blue and snaps down the front and around the bulgy diaper.

Little Matthew is getting the sleep he didn't get during the night. Ellie lays him down carefully in the crook of the leather chair and comes to stand near the kitchen island.

They had arrived late evening yesterday, the Tuesday before Thanksgiving. Suzan was taken back to the time of her own babies during the night when she heard Matthew's crying. She had offered to relieve Maddy, but Maddy said no.

"Maddy has had a time of it," Ellie says. When I take a leave of absence, it will be my turn to be up all hours. Over our time here we'll switch off. I don't have Maddy's touch."

"I can help. Ellie, when you look back on it, the time will have zipped by. He should get into a schedule soon."

"He travelled so well. Thank God."

Suzan has fallen in love. When she holds Matthew, she aches for Da and Matthew, her son. She feels that familiar physical tug in her breasts that nursing mothers feel, a sensation she never thought she would feel again. What better way to heal from her loss than with a baby in her arms? She nuzzles his neck as she holds him. Buying the crib was exactly the right thing to do. She wants them to come often in the coming years. It will fit in the gallery apartment as well. In fact, one might need two, one for downstairs and one for up.

Belle Haven has become foremost in her thinking. "There's nothing more I can do, Ellie, to keep Belle Haven. With Matthew part of the family, it is all the more important to me. I want to leave it to you someday."

"Mom, I can't believe Paul feels so strongly about having you move out, especially with Daan coming out here for school. Have you thought of showing him Da's last letter? Maybe he already suspects that you were more than friends before his mother died."

"You and Maddy are the only ones I've told about Da and me. The price of showing him the letter would be too high. I wouldn't be true to Da if I were to prove to them their father's intentions for me to live on here. I've nothing else in writing. Right now, I want to enjoy every minute we have here. I want Thursday to go well. Frank is confident the ceremony will come off without a hitch. Will you help with the pies tomorrow? I like cream better than canned milk in the pumpkin. There's just a subtle difference."

"Did you like being in the gallery?" Ellie says.

"Yes, very much. If I buy the gallery and am able to keep Belle Haven, would you consider moving here? The apartment would be just right for you three."

Ellie gets up from her chair and comes back to the kitchen. "Are you serious? She says, "Wow. One of us would have to get a job. I suppose it would be me. Maddy is such a natural at this mothering. We'd love to live outside the city. It was a great place to live as a single person, but having Maddy and Matt has brought its challenges. We're both worn out, and we've quarreled about daycare. We've even quarreled about which brand of diapers to buy."

"Things will get better. Maddy probably needs to get back to work."

Without any forethought, Suzan says, "The gallery makes enough to live on, plus I think business will get even better over time. I'd like to run it."

"Wow, Mom. Do you realize what you're proposing?

"I want to live here with all of my memories of Da. I want it to be a place where everyone can gather. Listen, I still have a key to the gallery, and Samantha won't be back until tomorrow evening. We have time to go down and look around. See what you think. I could teach a few students and carry on with my painting. Ellie, more than ever, it settles me to paint."

"Maddy would be thrilled," Ellie says. "We're finding the inner city isn't the best environment for daycare or school. Plus, we can't make it on one salary in the city. At some point if we stay, we'll have to use private schools, which are prohibitively expensive. There's a Sovereign Bank near here, a small branch in Lincoln City, maybe if I were willing to start at the entry level, they'd have a place for me."

"When is Paul's family getting here?"

"They'll be in tomorrow sometime before noon." Suzan says.

Tiny Matthew squirms and makes a sound. Ellie is there in an instant, tending to him, glancing at her watch. Suzan warms the bottle in the microwave for exactly ten seconds and shakes it well, taking it to Ellie who's in the process of changing a diaper. Ellie settles in to feed him. His eyes still closed, he sucks loudly, and they both are touched by his eagerness. With such a long torso, he'll be tall.

Ellie looks serene and beautiful, and Suzan will capture her profile in a painting after everyone leaves. She'll paint in a fully engorged breast rather than the blue oxford shirt she is wearing now. Only a touch of the pink aureole will be visible. Another young mother will buy it during the Christmas season.

When Maddy wakens, she looks disheveled. Her red hair seems to spring from all angles. When she hears the idea of living here and living outside the city, she agrees readily.

"Let's explore the idea. I think I could develop a private practice here. When can we go see? I've only been once, and all I remember is the beautiful art that surrounded us. Why does Samantha want to sell?"

"Let me call the realtor in case he's showing it."

In the car seat, Matthew opens his eyes and smiles a half smile. "You little charmer, keeping me up at night," Maddy says. Unintentionally, he blows milky bubbles.

When Suzan turns the key, the paint, the thinner and the linseed oil smell like a second home to her. Ellie and Maddy explore the upstairs. Maddy calls down, "It's much bigger than our apartment in San Francisco. I love the kitchen."

"How much do you think it would cost us to rent it from you, Mom?"

"In name, I could run it and possibly you could cover the mortgage. Shall I call the realtor and see what he thinks would be a fair offer?" Suzan shifts the baby to her other arm and dials the phone.

They make an appointment to meet him on Friday after Thanksgiving. Maddy and Ellie are locked arm in arm coming down the stairs.

Limited visibility

Wednesday, when Paul and his family arrive, the weather is blustery, with little visibility. Though they go to the window, the cove is hidden by a curtain of low-hanging fog and light, constant rain. Teri stays behind while Paul takes Daan and Charlotte to see where their grandfather died. They each don a rain jacket from the back entry, Paul in one of Da's yellow slickers.

Once on the bluff, Teri, Ellie, Maddy and Suzan can see them moving bulkily, enshrouded in mist. The rain, rarely a squall, has become a slow drizzle as they move up to and down from the cove. Paul has bent over the rock Suzan intends to move. The children join him and circle it, looking under it, standing on top. Daan picks up a small rock and examines it, then tosses it with a strong arm into the sea. Small changes we make to our world.

Her hood up, Charlotte sits on the ledge, leaning back on her elbows. *Truly, they are like native Oregonians, not minding the fog and rain,* Suzan thinks. *Where are their thoughts?* she wonders. Paul must be thinking about the major changes in his life: his father's death, his first child going off to college soon. Surely, he gives some credit to her for the many memories made here.

Charlotte, fully grown at fifteen, returns alone, tears on her cold cheeks. Suzan helps her in the jacket room where they keep a towel. Suzan and she embrace. "I know how you loved him," Suzan says.

"He even helped me with my geometry over the phone," Charlotte says. "He called me Charlie. He taught me how to cast the fishing line out far enough, but he still put that awful bait on for me. Oh, Grandma, if he had to die I wish he had died in his chair in the library instead of out in the cove."

Daan comes in, his feelings masked. He doesn't speak. Suzan stretches out the jackets to dry. He makes a fire, kneeling and blowing on it to get it started.

Paul stays out, looking out to sea without moving. Suzan sees his stance, his wide shoulders, and legs planted apart. In the opaque light, the shape of his figure is like Da. Suzan feels pulled toward him, wanting to console and ease his ache for his father's presence.

Da would be happy to have heard the news about his namesake grandson coming to Oregon next summer and possibly for four to six years after that. She's sure there would have been some nice wheels provided for him to make the trips back and forth to Coos Bay, Eugene and Belle Haven.

Thanksgiving morning, the sun hasn't risen. For an autumn morning, only a light mist hovers over the lawn and the flat, rocky terrain leading to the cove. Already the mist ascends, leaving droplets on the blades of the small yard of grass. Birds from the mountain forest herald the day has begun.

Suzan serves coffee to the crew of five who stand waiting in the windowed porch, looking out on the task ahead. The loggers wear oiled leather boots and pants cut off just above them. Their shirts are fresh as are their suspenders. Their knitted cotton undershirts extend beyond their sleeves.

They have twenty minutes before the first high tide after the incipient dawn at 7:26 a.m. The lumberjacks will use crowbars. Frank's crew plus Paul will pull the mast down with the knotted robes, hand over fist, using their combined weight until the rock gives. Much depends on the strength of the men with the crowbars to lift the front edges so the rock doesn't snag on the rough ground.

To prepare, Frank has put the mast in place. They have succeeded in getting it near the middle of the underbelly of the rock. A rock fulcrum has been shoved under the mast. They have excavated around the perimeter with pick axes, especially at the edges nearest the cove to make a downward sloping ramp. The giant puzzle piece now looks even more like the shape of the cove. The rusty black of the rock contrasts with the sand below.

Crowbars will be used to wedge and pries the great weight at the moment the mast is pulled toward the ground and the puzzle-shaped rock is released to slide into the cove. Frank has threaded four knotted ropes through an iron eye at the end of the mast with which to pull it down. Daan will count down. They must back quickly away from the mast as soon as the rock begins to slide. Frank projects that the long heavy spruce mast will fall back to the ground and roll. They have set up a perimeter of old tires to stop it.

Frank expects some of the surface under the loggers with the crowbars to cave away. He instructs them to jump to the sand below, staying clear of where the rock should land.

Guests are guided by Daan and Charlotte to the chairs placed in the shadowed space under the deck where they can easily see down the slope when the memorial rock is displaced. Each has been given a folded card. Da's smile is inside and the date of his birth and death.

Rosie putters indoors, arranging her fresh pastries in tempting mounds. She has guessed correctly, there are twenty-five to serve. She has generously counted two pastries per person, and the room smells like her bakery, yeasty and sweet.

Matthew sleeps on into the morning. Having been up in the night, Maddy would like to continue sleeping but rouses herself when Ellie stirs.

Assembling as a family, Paul, Teri, Daan and Charlotte take the front chairs, leaving a chair for Suzan and another for Ellie and Maddy. Suzan comes down just before the crew gets in place.

The maturing day will be clear, and the sun begins to brim with hope. In orange glory, the sun comes over the rim of their "half mountain".

Paul moves forward, his head down as he walks to become part of the crew. He turns, lifts his head and faces the group.

Clearing his throat, he says, "We buried my father in Maryland, but his spirit is still alive here at Belle Haven. For Suzan, Ellie, Maddy and the family, we want this rock to be a memorial to his love for Suzan and Belle Haven and for us all."

Daan begins the countdown after Frank checks his watch and gives him the nod. Instead of sitting, the group of friends and family stand.

At zero, all the team's efforts combine; the rock moves slowly, then slides into place an instant later. The rush of the tide washes over it in an entirely new pattern, in a fountain of spray, turning the memorial stone the color of waxed ebony. In the momentary quiet, they hear great sighs as the ocean sustains its rhythm. Then the men on the beach lift their crow bars in celebration. The standing audience applauds, and they extend themselves to embrace other members of the family.

The loggers return to their truck and bring the cast iron bench to be anchored later. They place it solidly on the new ledge. Da and Suzan's names are there. There are no dates except for the present: November 23, 2000. Because of Da, Belle Haven's shoreline is changed, perhaps forever, and Suzan rests.

After the event when everyone crowds inside for brunch, Paul wanders into Suzan's studio. He stoops to look more closely at the signature and date of the painting loved by his father. It dates prior to their marriage. The painting has obviously been painted from the place he stands, looking out to the sea. On the horizon is a cloud the size of a man's hand, like God's promise of rain to the Israelites. He goes to stand in front of the fire.

"Good fire, Daan, but then I'd expect that from an Eagle Scout."

He sits down in his father's chair, as if he's trying it out. He leans forward; he pushes back; he swivels once very slowly. After a time, he gets up and goes to the wall of books. He props the ladder against the shelves and reaches to the top for a large worn atlas of the world. Its cover is the color of dried grass. He spreads the thin book on the library table. With its fold-out pages worn in the creases, the binding beginning to fail, it looks like a throw-away. The pages are fragile, and the yellowed waxed sheets between them rustle as he carefully turns the pages, studying the penciled margins indicating where his father had traveled.

He calls to Daan, and they lean in together and study the maps. Paul shows him Java, Indonesia where Daan's grandfather was born, the Netherlands where he was raised, Kenya, Hawaii. From the margins, they read aloud the dates and the cities where he worked or visited. They find where they were born. The pencil lead has smudged in many places, and only traces remain.

"Unbelievable," Paul says, shaking his head. To Suzan, he says, "When we were kids he wrote us all the time from where his travels took him. Those letters could have made a book."

"He was special in that regard," Suzan says.

Daan goes outside to carry more wood in. Paul turns another page of the large atlas to the continent of Africa. There's more writing in the margin. In faint pencil, an asterisk by Abijan, Côte d'Ivoire leads to script slightly smudged over in the margin: *February 1970, met Suze.*

Paul fishes in his pocket, feeling of the ring he removed from his father's hand before the burial, intending to return it to Suzan. He turns it slowly. He reads the inscription.

A SEASON OF MISTS

Paul struggles with the information. Knowing he was conceived during the war before his parents married, he has long wondered about their lack of affection for each other, whether they were forced to marry though they didn't love each other. They always spoke to each other in their first language. Paul was never misled, but he had no insight into his parents' relationship, how it came to be or why it lacked intimacy. His mother was never able to speak fluent English, although she could read, and she could write . By the time he questioned their relationship in his mind, it was time for college at Berkley.

He looks at Suzan with new eyes. His father was happy here, happy with her. As a couple, they go back to 1970. The painting goes back to 1986.

When Paul married Teri, someone vibrant who loved life, he knew the power their love has over him. Perhaps his father had found a person who was like Teri is to him: loving, accepting, physically responsive. Paul had never witnessed his parents show any affection.

The pieces come together in his mind, and a major part of his father and Suzan's story falls in place for him.

"I believe you should have this," he says, stepping toward her, handing her the ring. The diamonds' quality is reflected by the strong sunlight coming through the skylights before she transfers the ring to her pocket. She notes that he has read the inscription. It was her last act. She had meant for it to go with Da's body.

"I've loved him for so long," she says.

He finds the pencil with the smudged erasure by the phone and gently cleans it against a note pad. Beckoning Suzan, he erases the faint asterisk near Abidjan and the information it conveys. He brushes the crackling page, and blows away the residue.

"I know that now. Thirty years?" Paul shifts. "Do we have an understanding?"

Suzan touches the back of his hand as it stays on the page, his finger near Abidjan where the erasure of the note in the margin means she can retain her privacy.

"Yes, we do."

Paul nods.

"How long would you want to live here if it were an option?"

"All my life," she whispers.

"Yes," he nods.

231

MYRNA BROWN

"To Autumn"

Season of mists and mellow fruitfulness
Close bosom-friend of the maturing sun
Conspiring with him how to load and bless
With fruit the vines that round the thatch-eves run;
To bend with apples the moss'd cottage-trees,
And fill all fruit with ripeness to the core;
To swell the gourd, and plump the hazel shells
With a sweet kernel; to set budding more,
And still more, later flowers for the bees,
Until they think warm days will never cease,
For Summer has o'er-brimm'd their clammy cells.

Who hath not seen thee oft amid thy store?
Sometimes whoever seeks abroad may find
Thee sitting careless on a granary floor,
Thy hair soft-lifted by the winnowing wind;
Or on a half-reap'd furrow sound asleep,
Drows'd with the fume of poppies, while thy hook
Spares the next swath and all its twined flowers:
And sometimes like a gleaner thou dost keep
Steady thy laden head across a brook;
Or by a cider-press, with patient look,
Thou watchest the last oozings hours by hours.

A SEASON OF MISTS

Where are the songs of Spring? Ay, where are they?
Think not of them, thou hast thy music too,-
While barred clouds bloom the soft-dying day,
And touch the stubble-plains with rosy hue;
Then in a wailful choir the small gnats mourn
Among the river swallows, borne aloft
Or sinking as the light wind lives or dies;
And full-grown lambs loud bleat from hilly bourn;
Hedge-crickets sing; and now with treble soft
The red-breast whistles from a garden-croft;
And gathering swallows twitter in the skies.

By John Keats
September 1819

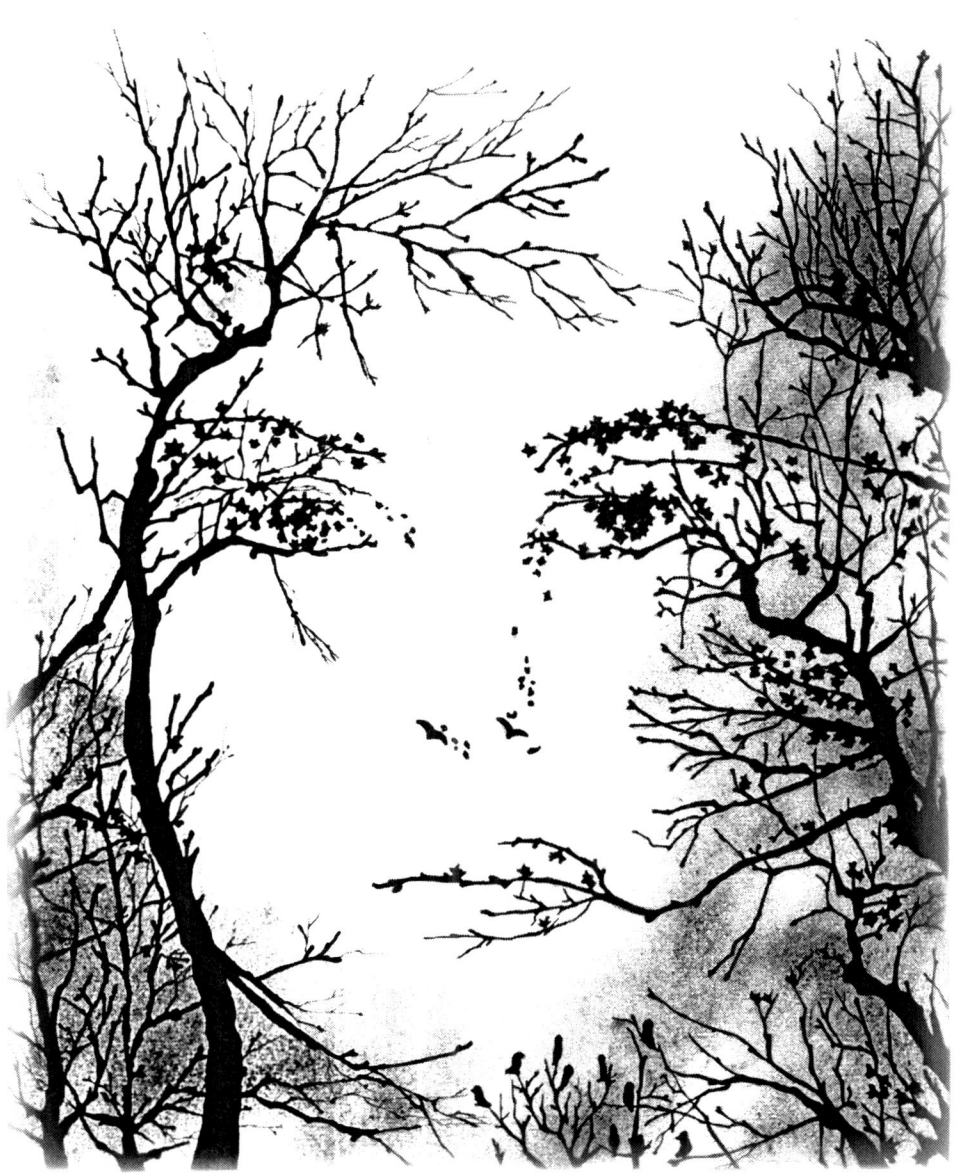

CPSIA information can be obtained
at www.ICGtesting.com
Printed in the USA
FFOW04n1913010816
26356FF